# *The* ENDOMORPH DIET

## Balanced and Delicious Recipes for Enhanced Metabolism and Lifelong Health for Endomorph Body Types with 28-Day Meal Plan

### MARY EDWARDS

**Warning-Disclaimer**

The purpose of this book is to educate and entertain. The author or publisher does not guarantee that anyone following the techniques, suggestions, tips, ideas, or strategies will become successful. The author and publisher shall have either liability or responsibility to anyone with respect to any loss or damage caused, or alleged to be caused, directly or indirectly by the information contained in this book.

# TABLE OF CONTENTS


**INTRODUCTION** 5

What is an Endomorph? 6

What is an Endomorph Diet? 6

How Does an Endomorph Diet Work? 6

What are health benefits of an Endomorph Diet? 7

How to do an Endomorph Diet? 8

Foods to Eat on an Endomorph Diet 8

Foods to Avoid on an Endomorph Diet 9

**CHAPTER 1: BREAKFAST RECIPES** 10

1. Hard-Boiled Eggs with Avocado Toast 10

2. Peanut Butter and Banana Sandwich 11

3. Banana Bread Muffins 11

4. Breakfast Salad 12

5. Oatmeal with Protein Powder 13

6. Breakfast Burrito 14

7. Hash Browns with Eggs 15

8. Breakfast Smoothie 16

9. Keto Waffles 16

10. Protein Pancakes 17

11. Cottage Cheese with Fruit and Honey 18

12. Scrambled Eggs with Black Beans and Salsa 19

13. Egg White Frittata 20

14. Greek Yogurt with Berries and Nuts 21

15. Sweet Potato Pancakes 21

16. Apple Cinnamon Oatmeal 22

17. Avocado Toast 23

18. Superfood Breakfast Bowl 24

19. Greek Egg Scramble 25

20. Avocado & Egg Toast 26

21. Banana Pancakes 27

22. Breakfast Bake 28

23. Pumpkin Pancakes 29

24. Asparagus and Swiss cheese Frittata 30

25. Maple Pecan Banana Muffins 31

26. Clean Protein Power Bars 32

27. Egg and Cheese Muffins 33

28. Cherry Protein Porridge 34

29. Chocolate Banana Protein Pancakes 35

30. Homemade Scallion Hash Brown Cakes 36

**CHAPTER 2: PASTA AND SOUPS** 37

1. Lentil Soup 37

2. Vegetable Soup 38

3. Lentil Stew 39

4. Artichoke and Olive Pasta 40

5. Vegetable Pasta 41

6. High-Protein Spaghetti 42

7. Muscle Lentil Soup 43

8. Mediterranean Shrimp Penne 44

9. Whole Wheat Pasta with Marinara Sauce 45

10. Quick Ramen with Shredded Chicken 46

11. Traditional Shrimp Scampi 47

12. Sweet Potato & Green Pea Soup 48

13. Bell Pasta with Kidney Beans 49

14. Farfalle with Chicken and Pesto 50

15. Spicy Buffalo Macaroni and Cheese 51

16. Cream of Broccoli Soup 52

**CHAPTER 3: BEEF, PORK, AND POULTRY** 53

1. Beef Shish Kebabs 53

2. Classic Steak 54

3. Lemon-Herb Grilled Chicken Salad 55

4. Pork Loin with Baked Apples 56

5. Japanese Steak Curry 57

6. Low-Fat Chicken Bacon Ranch Sandwich 58

7. Macro Roast Beef 59

8. Chicken Chili 60

9. Chicken Kabobs 61

10. Chicken Stir-Fry 62

11. Salad with Grilled Chicken 63

12. Roasted Balsamic Chicken 64

13. Spicy Turkey Stir Fry 65

14. Pulled Chicken BBQ Sandwich 66

15. Grilled Chicken Breast Sandwich 67

16. Teriyaki Chicken with Jasmine Rice 68

17. Grilled Chicken Breast with Roasted Vegetables 69

18. Olive Chicken 70

## CHAPTER 4: FISH AND SEAFOOD    71

1. Avocado and Salmon Salad    71
2. Rustic Scallops with Coriander and Lime    72
3. Shrimp Shiitake Pot Stickers    73
4. Protein-Packed Paella    74
5. Grilled Tuna Teriyaki    75
6. Tuna Salad Sandwich on Whole-Wheat Bread    76
7. Salmon with Quinoa and Roasted Veggies    77
8. Parmesan-Crusted Salmon    78
9. Garlic and Herb Seared Salmon    79
10. Shrimp Creole    80
11. Super Human Sea Bass with Sizzling Spices    81
12. Bourbon Lime Salmon    82
13. Brawny Baked Haddock with Spinach    83
14. Tangy Trout    84
15. Cod with Bacon, Red Onion, and Kale    85
16. Lemon Dill Salmon    86
17. Healthy Fish and Chips    87
18. Sea Bass with Vegetables    88

## CHAPTER 5: SIDES AND SALADS    89

1. Salmon Chickpea Salad    89
2. Cabbage Slaw    90
3. Shrimp Taco Salad    91
4. Italian Pasta Salad    92
5. Red Onion and Olive Focaccia    93
6. Summer Squash Casserole    94
7. Roasted Butternut Squash    95
8. Stuffed Mushrooms    95
9. Italian Tuna Salad    96
10. Avocado and Tuna Salad    97
11. Garlic Parmesan Fries    98
12. Cilantro Lime Low-Carb Rice    99
13. Citrus Spinach    100
14. Vegetarian Cakes    101
15. Curried Chickpea Salad    102
16. Lentil and Feta Tabbouleh    103
17. Garlic Mashed Sweet Potatoes    104

## CHAPTER 6: DESSERTS    105

1. Cinnamon Protein Apple Slices    105
2. Triple Berry Yogurt Parfait    106
3. Frozen Chocolate Banana    107
4. Protein Sludge    108
5. Apple Crisp    108
6. Paleo Brownies    109
7. Keto Cheesecake    110
8. Frozen Banana Yogurt Bark    111
9. No-Bake Cookie Bites    112
10. Almond Cookies    113
11. Apple Oatmeal Crunchy    114
12. Chocolate Banana Cups    115
13. Apple Pie Bars    116
14. Cinnamon Apple Protein Bars    117
15. Peanut Butter Protein Cookies    118
16. Café Mocha Protein Bars    119
17. High-Protein Oatmeal Cookies    120
18. Greek Yogurt Parfait    121
19. Vegan Chocolate Chip Cookies    122
20. Strawberry Shortcake    123

## CHAPTER 7: SMOOTHIE RECIPES    124

1. Peanut Butter & Banana Smoothie    124
2. Oatmeal & Berry Smoothie    125
3. Tropical Smoothie    126
4. Peanut Butter & Jelly Smoothie    127
5. Avocado Smoothie    128
6. Green Machine Smoothie    129
7. Keto Smoothie    130
8. Spinach Smoothie    131
9. Mango Smoothie    132
10. Chocolate Peanut Butter Cup Smoothie    133
11. Chocolate Smoothie    134
12. Green Apple Smoothie    135
13. Chocolate Banana Smoothie    136
14. Berry Blast Smoothie    137

## 28 DAYS MEAL PLAN    138

# INTRODUCTION

The "Endomorph Diet Cookbook" is a culinary adventure created for people with endomorphic bodies. This book goes beyond just a set of formulas; it acts as a manual that will help you accept an eating style that supports your natural body constitution, improves your metabolic processes, and helps achieve the desired wellness goals.

Because this body type is inclined to store both muscle and fat quickly, there are specific ways of feeding it. As such, we have developed a range of recipes that conform to the principles of an endomorph diet, balanced macronutrient ratios, whole foods-based menus and emphasis on insulin sensitivity or metabolic health.

The numerous categories of meals from which one can choose, such as morning energy boosters, healthy lunches for busy days at work, sumptuous dinners and light snacks, among others, are contained in the book. Each recipe considers the ratio of proteins' fats' and carbohydrates, besides having higher fiber content and lower sugar levels required for maintaining weight issues vis-a-vis energy-boosting purposes.

However, this cookbook isn't only about food; it's about embracing your body shape. It's understanding that there is no one-size-fits-all way to health. We want each dish to feed your system and make you fall in love with cooking while bringing awareness about how good food choices impact our overall well-being.

It's worth noting that endomorphs tend to retain more body fat than other body types, meaning they need proper diets and nutrition for healthy living. If you want an advanced method towards finding out what kind of diet suits your individual needs best, following a nutritional regime for your particular type could be used to capitalize on its strengths and thus compensate for its weaknesses.

Though not heavily researched compared to other diets, much data supports this concept. In particular, endomorph diet plans are based around whole foods, which provide all the essential nutrients if there is a balance between macronutrients and other healthier food groups, with no group being omitted.

# What is an Endomorph?

There are three main body types under this framework: mesomorph, ectomorph and endomorph. Mesomorphs naturally have muscular and strong bodies with a male inverted triangle or female hourglass figure. People with this kind of body type generally have high metabolism rates and low percentage fat content.

Ectomorphs are usually tall and thin with long arms and legs, coupled with an inborn rapid rate of metabolism. They maintain their weight without much ado; thus, they may eat more without worrying about gaining weight and even find it challenging to gain pounds.

Endomorphs usually carry higher body fats as well as lower metabolisms. "Endomorphic individuals face difficulties in shedding off their weights because of increased biological tendencies of having much fat," says Lauren Chaunt, registered dietitian nutritionist. "They are generally characterized by slow metabolic processes that make them prone to putting on few pounds."

## What is an Endomorph Diet?

The endomorph diet comprises a tailored and efficient method of losing weight for people who consider themselves endomorphs; it is used by individuals identified as endomorphs. This dietary approach focuses on lean proteins, complex carbohydrates, and healthy fats to optimize metabolism, promote muscle development, and manage body composition. In addition to making smart food choices, portion control is vital for endomorphs because they need to regulate their eating habits to avoid excessive intake.

## How Does an Endomorph Diet Work?

People can cut out some food and increase the intake of other nutrients to focus on reducing overall caloric intake for the endomorph diet. People might start eating less carbs and protein more healthily, as well as healthy omega-3 fatty acids.

"A diet comprising of nutrient-dense foods such as lean quality protein, complex carbohydrates and healthy fats," says Chaunt, "is recommended for people having an endomorphic body type." Usually, individuals with this kind of body type may need a meal plan that incorporates unrefined high-fiber foods and healthy fats, proteins, fruits, vegetables and carbohydrates in their diets.

# What are health benefits of an Endomorph Diet?

Endomorph Diet has several advantages, such as losing weight and avoiding fat build-up. The benefits of an endomorph diet include reduced risk of cardiovascular diseases, reduced blood pressure and boosted skin health.

**Weight Management:** Losing body fat is possible through the endomorph diet when one takes macronutrients in a balanced manner but with fewer carbohydrates. Its primary emphasis on protein and fiber increases satiety and prevents overconsumption, which makes this even better.

**Improved Insulin Sensitivity:** Insulin sensitivity in endomorphs tends to be higher. A low-sugar processed carbohydrate diet helps to maintain sugar levels, thus lowering the chances of insulin resistance, which often precedes type 2 diabetes.

**Enhanced Metabolism:** Instead of aiding muscle growth only, proteins increase metabolic rate because digestion requires higher energy than fats or carbohydrates.

**Reduced Risk for Cardiovascular Diseases:** By cutting out processed foods high in sugars and introducing healthy fats into our meals, this Diet enhances heart health. It manages cholesterol levels, thus decreasing hypertension and other related cardiac problems.

**Better Digestive Health:** For regular bowel movements and preventing ailments like constipation, an abundant amount of dietary fiber from whole grains, fruits/vegetables ensures a healthier digestive system.

**Increased Energy Levels:** Maintaining alertness and avoiding spike-and-crash episodes associated with high sugar/high refined carbs diets are reasons one should consume balanced meals containing adequate amounts of protein, fat, and complex carbohydrates.

**Overall Nutritional Balance:** Incorporating different food groups guarantees the proper intake of essential vitamins and minerals, including antioxidants, ensuring good nutrition according to Endomorph Diet's principles.

**Mental Health Benefits:** In addition to improved mood and cognitive function brought about by balanced blood sugar levels due to eating nutritious foods.

# How to do an Endomorph Diet?

The amount of calories eaten on a meal plan for an endomorph will depend on the basal metabolic rate and your activity level. An endomorph diet should have 40% of its calories from protein, 40% from fats and 20% from carbohydrates. For instance, people who need to lose weight should reduce their daily calorie intake by 300-500.

The duration within which one is advised to eat an endomorph diet may differ because people have different goals and health conditions. If eating this type of food reduces body fat levels and improves overall health, they can consume low-carb meals.

There are several recommendations to be observed while on an endomorph diet. People should stick to complex carbohydrate foods rather than simple ones. In addition, it is better to consume healthy protein sources like heart-healthy fish, organic chicken, and lean cuts of red meat. Finally, people following an endomorph diet should only eat low-carb fruits like melons.

# Foods to Eat on an Endomorph Diet

An endomorph diet allows for the consumption of certain types of food. Have a look at the endomorph diet food list.

**Protein-rich Foods:** Chicken, turkey, fish, eggs, and plant-based proteins such as lentils and chickpeas have high protein content, enabling muscle growth while keeping you full.

**Low-Glycemic Carbohydrates:** Examples like quinoa, brown rice, oats and sweet potatoes are good sources of energy that do not lead to sudden increases in blood sugar levels.

**Fiber-Rich Vegetables** include leafy greens, broccoli, cauliflower and other non-starchy vegetables. They aid in digestion and also help to keep one full.

**Healthy Fats:** These are avocados, nuts, seeds, and olive oil, crucial to maintaining hormonal balance and thus making it easier to feel content.

**Moderate Fruit Intake:** For example, berries, apples, and pears contain less sugar but more fiber.

# Foods to Avoid on an Endomorph Diet

People should avoid certain foods while following the endomorph diet.

**Refined carbohydrates:** Sugar-loaded processed foods like white bread and pastries lack nutrients.

**Sugary snacks and drinks:** For instance, these include confectioneries, sodas, and high-sugar juices, which may result in an instant rise in blood sugar levels and weight increase.

**High-fat meats:** Like fatty pieces of pork or beef and sausages or bacon that contain massive amounts of unwanted fat and calories.

**Fried Foods:** Including French fries and fried chicken, which are usually packed with high-calorie content and unhealthy fats.

**High-sodium foods** include fast food joints, canned soups, and processed snacks. Too much sodium can cause water retention hence bloating.

## 1. Hard-Boiled Eggs with Avocado Toast

**Prep Time: 10 minutes Cook Time: 12 minutes Servings: 1**

### Ingredients

- 2 large eggs
- 1 ripe avocado
- 2 slices of whole-grain bread
- Salt and pepper, to taste
- Optional: a sprinkle of chili flakes or paprika, fresh herbs, or a squeeze of lemon juice

### Instructions

1. Put eggs into a pot and cover them with cold water by one inch. Bring the water over medium-high heat to boil. As soon as it starts boiling, place a lid on the pan and remove it from the stove. After 12 minutes, move the eggs to a bowl of icy cold water.
2. Meanwhile, carve and remove the pit from the avocado. Scoop out the pulp in a bowl and mash it. Add salt, pepper, and, if desired, some lemon juice.
3. Toast slices of whole wheat bread until they are crispy enough for you.
4. Evenly spread the mashed avocado on each slice of toast. Remove shells from cooled hard-boiled eggs, then chop or slice them and put them on top of mashed avocado.
5. Garnish with a pinch of chili flakes, paprika, or fresh herbs for more flavor, according to your preference. Adjust salt and pepper to taste.

**Nutrition (per serving):**

Calories: 450 kcal Protein: 20 g Carbohydrates: 35 g Fiber: 15 g Healthy Fats: 25 g

# 2. Peanut Butter and Banana Sandwich

**Prep Time: 5 minutes Cook Time: 0 minutes Servings: 1**

## Ingredients

- 2 slices of whole-grain bread
- 2 tbsp natural peanut butter
- 1 medium banana, sliced
- Optional: a sprinkle of cinnamon

## Instructions

1. If you want to, toast the whole-wheat bread slices for as long as you like until they become hard and crunchy.
2. Now spread the peanut butter smoothly on one side of every piece of toasted bread.
3. On top of the peanut butter, lay the banana slabs on one slice. A little cinnamon or honey can be sprinkled onto it if desired.
4. Close this sandwich with the other slice of bread with its underside covered with peanut butter.

**Nutrition (per serving):**

Calories: 430 kcal Protein: 15 g Carbohydrates: 50 g Fiber: 8 g Healthy Fats: 20 g

# 3. Banana Bread Muffins

**Prep Time: 15 minutes Cook Time: 25 minutes Servings: 12 muffins**

## Ingredients

- 1 ¾ cups of whole wheat flour or almond flour
- 1 tsp baking soda
- ½ tsp salt
- 1/3 cup of melted coconut oil
- ½ cup of honey or maple syrup
- 2 eggs at room temperature
- 1 cup of mashed ripe bananas
- ¼ cup of milk
- 1 tsp vanilla extract
- Optional: ½ cup of walnuts or pecans (chopped), dark chocolate chips, or blueberries

## Instructions

1. Preheat your oven to 325°F. Grease a 12-cup of a muffin tin or line it with muffin cups.
2. Whisk flour, baking soda, and salt in a large bowl.
3. In another bowl, stir melted coconut oil (or applesauce), honey or maple syrup. Add eggs and beat well; add mashed bananas, milk, and vanilla extract.
4. Pour wet ingredients into dry ones and mix with a spoon or spatula until the batter is combined. Be careful not to overmix! If desired, fold nuts, chocolate chips or blueberries.
5. Divide the batter evenly among the cups of your muffin tin. You may also wish to sprinkle tops with a few extra nuts or chips.
6. Bake for 20-25 minutes; test if it is done by inserting a toothpick in one of the muffins; check if it will come out clean.
7. Allow muffins to cool for about 5 minutes in the pan before transferring them to a wire rack for complete cooling.

### Nutrition (per muffin)

Calories: 200 kcal Protein: 4 g Carbohydrates: 30 g Fiber: 4 g Healthy Fats: 9 g

# 4. Breakfast Salad

**Prep Time: 15 minutes Cook Time: 5 minutes Servings: 1**

## Ingredients

- 2 cups of mixed greens
- 1 hard-boiled egg, sliced
- ½ avocado, sliced
- ¼ cup of cherry tomatoes, halved
- 2 tbsp crumbled feta cheese or goat cheese
- 2 slices of turkey bacon, cooked and crumbled
- 1 tbsp olive oil
- 1 tbsp balsamic vinegar
- Salt and pepper, to taste
- Optional: a sprinkle of seeds

## Instructions

1. Rinse mixed greens and chop if needed. Slice hardboiled egg and avocado. Cut cherry tomatoes in half. Cook turkey bacon till crispy, then crumble it.

2. Combine mixed greens; egg sliced hard-boiled, cut-up avocado, tomatoes cherry halved, crumbled turkey bacon and cheese in a large bowl.
3. Drizzle salad with olive oil and balsamic vinegar. Toss gently to combine. Season with salt and pepper according to your taste.
4. For variety in texture and nutrition, sprinkle any seeds or nuts of your choice on the salad.

**Nutrition (per serving):**

Calories: 400 kcal Protein: 20 g Carbohydrates: 20 g Fiber: 8 g Healthy Fats: 30 g

# 5. Oatmeal with Protein Powder

**Prep Time: 5 minutes Cook Time: 5 minutes Servings: 1**

## Ingredients

- ½ cup of rolled oats
- 1 cup of water or milk
- 1 scoop of your preferred protein powder
- ½ banana, sliced
- 1 tbsp almond butter
- Optional toppings: fresh berries, chia seeds, a sprinkle of cinnamon, or a drizzle of honey

## Instructions

1. Heat one cup of water or milk to boiling in a small saucepan. Put in rolled oats and turn down the heat for it to simmer. Cook for approximately 5 minutes, stirring occasionally, until oats are soft and have absorbed all liquid.
2. Take out the saucepan from the source of heat. Stir protein powder in it until well combined with oatmeal porridge. If the mixture is too dense, add more water or milk to bring it to your preferred thickness.
3. Move oatmeal to a bowl. Add sliced banana, almond/peanut butter and any other toppings that might be preferred.

**Nutrition (per serving)**

Calories: 350 kcal Protein: 30g Carbohydrates: 40g Fiber: 6g Healthy Fats: 10 g

# 6. Breakfast Burrito



## Ingredients

- 1 large whole-grain or low-carb tortilla
- 2 eggs
- ¼ cup of cooked black beans
- ¼ cup of bell peppers, diced
- ¼ cup of onion, diced
- 1 tbsp olive oil
- ¼ cup of shredded cheese
- 2 tbsp salsa
- Salt and pepper, to taste
- Optional: ¼ avocado, sliced; 2 tbsp Greek yogurt or sour cream

## Instructions

1. Heat olive oil in a skillet over medium heat. Add the diced bell peppers and onion, sautéing for 3-5 minutes until they become soft.
2. Beat the eggs and pour them into the skillet with the vegetables. Keep stirring until the eggs are fully cooked. Put salt and pepper to taste.
3. Warm the tortilla in a separate pan or microwave for 15-20 seconds to become softer.
4. Layer on the tortilla, scrambled egg and vegetable mix, black beans, cheese and salsa. If you have any, even avocado slices and Greek yogurt can be added if preferred.
5. Wrap the filled tortilla by folding its sides inwardly, then roll it tight.
6. Grill the burrito in a skillet for 2-3 minutes on each side to make it crispy outside.

**Nutrition (per serving):**

Calories: 500 kcal Protein: 25 g Carbohydrates: 45 g Fiber: 8 g Healthy Fats: 25 g

# 7. Hash Browns with Eggs

**Prep Time: 10 minutes Cook Time: 20 minutes Servings: 1**

## Ingredients

- 1 medium russet potato, grated
- 2 eggs
- 1 tbsp olive oil
- Salt and pepper, to taste
- Optional: ¼ cup of diced onions, ¼ cup of chopped bell peppers, 1 minced garlic clove

## Instructions

1. Peel and grate the potato. Put the grated potato on a clean towel or in a sieve to remove any moisture. This step is essential in making crispy hash browns.
2. Heat half of the olive oil in a nonstick pan over medium-high heat. Place grated potatoes in it and press them to form a thin layer. Cook for 5 minutes till golden brown and crispy at the bottom. Flip the other side and cook for an additional 5 minutes. Add salt and pepper to taste.
3. In another frying pan, pour the remaining olive oil and fry eggs according to your preference.
4. Put the cooked eggs on a plate on top of the crispy hash browns.

**Nutrition (per serving):**

Calories: 350 kcal Protein: 15 g Carbohydrates: 35 g Fiber: 5 g Healthy Fats: 20 g

# 8. Breakfast Smoothie

**Prep Time: 5 minutes Cook Time: 0 minutes Servings: 1**

## Ingredients

- 1 cup of unsweetened almond milk
- ½ banana, frozen
- ½ cup of mixed berries
- 1 scoop protein powder
- 1 tbsp chia seeds or flaxseeds
- 1 tbsp almond butter or peanut butter
- Optional: a handful of spinach or kale for extra nutrients
- Optional: a few ice cubes for a thicker texture

## Instructions

1. Combine the almond milk, frozen banana, mixed berries, protein powder, chia or flaxseeds and almond or peanut butter in a blender. Add spinach or kale if you want.
2. Add a few ice cubes for a thicker smoothie. Blend until it is smooth.
3. Pour the liquid into a glass and drink at once.

**Nutrition (per serving):**

Calories: 350 kcal Protein: 25 g Carbohydrates: 30 g Fiber: 8 g Healthy Fats: 15 g


# 9. Keto Waffles

**Prep Time: 10 minutes Cook Time: 5 minutes Servings: 2 waffles**

## Ingredients

- 1 cup of almond flour
- 2 tbsp erythritol
- 1 tsp baking powder
- 2 large eggs
- ¼ cup of unsweetened almond milk
- 2 tbsp melted butter or coconut oil
- 1 tsp vanilla extract
- Pinch of salt

# Instructions

1. Put almond flour, erythritol, baking powder, and salt in one container.
2. Beat eggs in a different bowl with almond milk, melted butter (or coconut oil), and vanilla extract.
3. You will get a smooth batter after mixing the wet ingredients with the dry ones.
4. Observe guidelines for preheating your waffle maker.
5. Place 50% of the mixture into the waffle maker and cook it for about five minutes or until it becomes golden brown and crispy as per the instructions supplied with an appliance.
6. Repeat with the second half of the batter.

### Nutrition (per waffle):

Calories: 400 kcal Protein: 15 g Carbohydrates: 12 g Fiber: 5 g Healthy Fats: 35 g

# 10. Protein Pancakes

**Prep Time: 10 minutes Cook Time: 5 minutes Servings: 2**

# Ingredients

- ½ cup of rolled oats
- 1 banana, ripe
- 2 large eggs
- 1 scoop protein powder
- ½ tsp baking powder
- ¼ cup of unsweetened almond milk
- ½ tsp vanilla extract
- Pinch of salt
- Cooking spray or a small amount of butter/coconut oil for the pan

# Instructions

1. Place the quick-cooking oats, a banana, two eggs, protein powder, baking powder, almond milk, vanilla extract and a pinch of salt into a blender. Blend until smooth.
2. Heat a nonstick skillet or griddle over medium heat. Lightly grease using cooking spray, butter or coconut oil.
3. Pour about ¼ cup of batter per pancake on the skillet. Cook until bubbles appear at the top, then flip and cook on the other side for one to two minutes until it becomes slightly brownish.

4. While still hot, serve with some toppings, such as fresh berries, Greek yogurt, and sugar-free syrup.

**Nutrition (per serving):**

Calories: 350 kcal Protein: 25 g Carbohydrates: 35 g Fiber: 6 g Healthy Fats: 10 g

# 11. Cottage Cheese with Fruit and Honey

**Prep Time: 5 minutes Cook Time: 0 minutes Servings: 1**

## Ingredients

- 1 cup of low-fat cottage cheese
- ½ cup of mixed fresh fruit
- 1 tbsp honey
- Optional: a sprinkle of cinnamon or chia seeds

## Instructions

1. Take a bowl and put the cottage cheese in it.
2. After that, spread the top of the cottage cheese with any fresh fruit you like.
3. Then drop some honey from above. Feel free to add as much honey as you prefer to your taste buds.
4. Finally, sprinkle cinnamon or chia seeds over the top for added flavor and nutrition.

**Nutrition (per serving):**

Calories: 300 kcal Protein: 30 g Carbohydrates: 35 g Fiber: 4 g Healthy Fats: 5 g

# 12. Scrambled Eggs with Black Beans and Salsa

**Prep Time: 5 minutes Cook Time: 10 minutes Servings: 1**

## Ingredients

- 2 large eggs
- ½ cup of canned black beans, rinsed and drained
- ¼ cup of salsa
- 1 tbsp olive oil or cooking spray
- Salt and pepper, to taste
- Optional: shredded cheese, diced avocado, chopped cilantro, or a squeeze of lime for extra flavor

## Instructions

1. Wash and drain the black beans. In a bowl, mix beaten eggs with salt and pepper.
2. Put the olive oil in a non-stick skillet heated over medium heat. In it, pour the beaten eggs. After they have sat, stir them gently until they are barely solidified and slightly liquid. Turn off the oven as they will still cook from its warmth alone.
3. Flash heat black beans quickly in another pan or the same one as above. This can be done before cooking the eggs if preferred.
4. Top with warmed black beans on a plate of scrambled eggs, then spoon salsa on top of all that.
5. Shredded cheese can be added, chopped cilantro, diced avocado, or lime juice squeezed onto it.

**Nutrition (per serving):**

Calories: 350 kcal Protein: 25 g Carbohydrates: 25 g Fiber: 8 g Healthy Fats: 20 g

# 13. Egg White Frittata

**Prep Time: 10 minutes Cook Time: 20 minutes Servings: 2**

## Ingredients

- 1 cup of egg whites
- 1 small zucchini, diced
- 1/2 bell pepper, diced
- 1/4 cup of diced onion
- 1/2 cup of spinach, chopped
- 1/4 cup of cherry tomatoes, halved
- 1/4 cup of low-fat feta cheese or goat cheese (optional)
- 1 tbsp olive oil
- Salt and pepper, to taste
- Optional herbs: basil, parsley, or chives

## Instructions

1. Preheat the oven to 375°F (190°C).
2. Begin by heating some olive oil in an oven-proof skillet, which is medium heated. Mix the zucchini, onion and bell pepper. Then, sauté them until they become soft but not too much.
3. Season your vegetables with salt and pepper, and pour the egg whites over them afterwards. Only cook for approximately 3-4 minutes, until cooked around the sides.
4. The next step is to sprinkle halved cherry tomatoes over your frittata (feta cheese optional).
5. The pan should be moved into the oven and then baked; it takes about ten minutes or fifteen to turn golden brown and look like a set frittata on top.
6. Then, let the frittata cool down for a little while before slicing it into individual servings; if you want, garnish each piece with fresh herbs like cilantro or parsley.

**Nutrition (per serving)**

Calories: 200 kcal Protein: 20 g Carbohydrates: 10 g Fiber: 2 g Healthy Fats: 10 g

# 14. Greek Yogurt with Berries and Nuts

**Prep Time: 5 minutes Cook Time: 0 minutes Servings: 1**

## Ingredients

- 1 cup of plain Greek yogurt
- ½ cup of mixed berries
- ¼ cup of mixed nuts, roughly chopped
- Optional: a drizzle of honey or a sprinkle of cinnamon for added flavor

## Instructions

1. Place the Greek yoghurt into a bowl.
2. Over the yoghurt, add a mixture of berries.
3. For the nut pieces of berry, shed over them.
4. If one needs to spice it up more, they can pour some honey or sprinkle cinnamon.

**Nutrition (per serving)**

Calories: 300 kcal Protein: 25 g Carbohydrates: 20 g Fiber: 5 g Healthy Fats: 15 g


# 15. Sweet Potato Pancakes

**Prep Time: 15 minutes Cook Time: 10 minutes Servings: 2**

## Ingredients

- 1 medium sweet potato
- 2 large eggs
- 1/2 cup of almond flour or whole wheat flour
- 1/4 cup of milk
- 1 tsp baking powder
- 1/2 tsp cinnamon
- 1/4 tsp nutmeg
- Pinch of salt
- Cooking spray or butter for the pan
- Optional: honey or maple syrup for serving

## Instructions

1. Prick the sweet potato using a fork and put it inside the microwave until tender, 5-7 minutes, or bake in the oven. After cooling down, peel and mash it.
2. Combine eggs, milk and mashed sweet potato in a bowl. Stir properly. Combine flour, cinnamon powder, nutmeg powder, and salt with baking powder in another bowl. Mix dry ingredients with wet ingredients by stirring them together just until combined.
3. Heat skillet over medium heat, then spray cooking oil or add butter. Drop ¼ cup of batter for each pancake. Cook until golden brown for 2-3 minutes on each side.
4. Serve these pancakes hot. Optionally, add several drops of honey or maple syrup to top them if desired.

### Nutrition (per serving)

Calories: 320 kcal Protein: 12 g Carbohydrates: 35 g Fiber: 6 g Healthy Fats: 16 g

# 16. Apple Cinnamon Oatmeal

**Prep Time: 5 minutes Cook Time: 10 minutes Servings: 1**

## Ingredients

- ½ cup of rolled oats
- 1 cup of water or milk
- 1 medium apple, peeled and diced
- 1 tsp cinnamon
- 1 tbsp chopped nuts
- Optional: 1 tbsp honey, A pinch of nutmeg

## Instructions

1. Bring water or milk to a boiling point in a saucepan. Add in rolled oats and reduce heat to simmer.
2. Add diced apple and cinnamon while stirring. Let it cook for another 5-7 minutes, occasionally stirring until the oatmeal becomes soft while the mixture is thickened.
3. Remove from heat when oatmeal is through cooking. Add some honey or syrup from maple for extra sweetness with nutmeg or ground ginger.
4. Serve the oatmeal in a bowl. Sprinkle with chopped nuts to add texture and nutrition.

### Nutrition (per serving)

Calories: 300 kcal Protein: 8 g Carbohydrates: 50 g Fiber: 8 g Healthy Fats: 6 g

# 17. Avocado Toast

**Prep Time: 5 minutes Cook Time: 3 minutes Servings: 1**

## Ingredients

- 1 ripe avocado
- 2 slices of whole-grain bread
- 1 tbsp lemon juice
- Salt and pepper, to taste
- Optional toppings: sliced tomatoes, radishes, sprouts, poached egg, sesame seeds, or chilli flakes

## Instructions

1. Put the slices of bread into a toaster or a frying pan over medium heat until they turn as crispy as you like.
2. As the bread gets toasted, halve the avocado, remove its seed and scoop the whole fruit into a bowl. Mash with a fork, leaving some lumps for texture while adding lemon juice, salt and pepper.
3. Apply an equal amount of mashed avocado onto all the pieces of toast.
4. You can also enhance the flavor and nutrition value by putting optional toppings on your dish such as chopped tomatoes, radishes, sprouts, poached eggs, sesame seeds or chili flakes if you wish to do so.

**Nutrition (per serving)**

Calories: 400 kcal Protein: 10 g Carbohydrates: 40 g Fiber: 15 g Healthy Fats: 25 g

# 18. Superfood Breakfast Bowl

**Prep Time: 10 minutes Cook Time: 0 minutes Servings: 1**

## Ingredients

- 1 cup of Greek yogurt
- ¼ cup of granola
- ½ banana, sliced
- ¼ cup of mixed berries
- 1 tbsp chia seeds
- 1 tbsp flaxseeds, ground
- 1 tbsp pumpkin seeds or sunflower seeds
- Optional: a drizzle of honey or a sprinkle of cinnamon for added flavor

## Instructions

1. In a bowl, add the Greek yoghurt as the base.
2. Add granola on top of the yogurt.
3. Top with banana slices and sliced mixed berries over the granola.
4. On top of these fruits go chia seeds, ground flaxseeds, and pumpkin or sunflower seeds.
5. If you wish to have a more pronounced taste, you can drizzle a little honey or sprinkle some cinnamon.

**Nutrition (per serving):**

Calories: 400 kcal Protein: 25 g Carbohydrates: 40 g Fiber: 8 g Healthy Fats: 15 g

# 19. Greek Egg Scramble

**Prep Time: 5 minutes Cook Time: 10 minutes Servings: 1**

## Ingredients

- 3 large eggs
- 1 tbsp olive oil
- ¼ cup of diced tomatoes
- ¼ cup of chopped spinach
- ¼ cup of crumbled feta cheese
- 2 tbsp diced red onion
- Salt and pepper, to taste
- Optional: a sprinkle of oregano or basil, black olives, or a drizzle of tzatziki sauce

## Instructions

1. Mix the eggs with salt and pepper in a bowl.
2. Heat the olive oil in a non-stick frying pan over medium heat. Meanwhile, cook the onions for a while till they become tender. Cook some spinach and diced tomatoes until the spinach turns soft.
3. Pour vegetables into a skillet, then pour in eggs that have been beaten and leave them for some time. Softly stir it up just before it is done when still soft.
4. Sprinkle feta cheese crumbs on top of the egg mix. Stir softly to blend everything.
5. Remove from heat. You can also sprinkle oregano/basil, black olives, or tzatziki sauce.

**Nutrition (per serving)**

Calories: 400 kcal Protein: 25 g Carbohydrates: 10 g Fiber: 2 g Healthy Fats: 30 g

# 20. Avocado & Egg Toast

**Prep Time: 5 minutes Cook Time: 5 minutes Servings: 1**

## Ingredients

- 1 ripe avocado
- 2 slices of whole-grain bread
- 2 eggs
- 1 tbsp olive oil or cooking spray
- Salt and pepper, to taste
- Optional toppings: chili flakes, fresh herbs, or a sprinkle of cheese

## Instructions

1. Start by putting the whole-grain bread slices in a toaster and set them to how crispy you want.
2. Cut the avocado into two halves as the bread is toasted, remove the pit, and transfer its flesh to a bowl. With your fork, mash the avocado as your salt and pepper it.
3. Put olive oil on a nonstick pan and put it over medium heat. Afterwards, place eggs into the skillet and cook according to your taste.
4. Apply even amounts of mashed avocado on each of these pieces of toast. They have been cooked, so lay those eggs gently on them.
5. If desired, sprinkle some chili flakes, herbs or cheese.

**Nutrition (per serving):**

Calories: 500 kcal Protein: 20 g Carbohydrates: 40 g Fiber: 15 g Healthy Fats: 30 g

# 21. Banana Pancakes

**Prep Time: 10 minutes Cook Time: 10 minutes Servings: 2**

## Ingredients

- 2 medium ripe bananas
- 2 large eggs
- 1/2 cup of oat flour
- 1/2 tsp baking powder
- 1/2 tsp cinnamon
- A pinch of salt
- Cooking spray or butter for the pan
- Optional: a few drops of vanilla extract
- Optional toppings: fresh berries, a drizzle of honey or maple syrup, yogurt, or nut butter

## Instructions

1. Put the bananas in a bowl and smash them with a fork until smooth.
2. Beat eggs and incorporate them into the squashed bananas, mixing well. If you want, add some vanilla extract.
3. Combine oat flour, baking powder, cinnamon, and salt.
4. Preheat a nonstick skillet over medium heat; coat it with cooking spray or butter. Pour about 1/4 cup of batter for each pancake. Cook for about two to three minutes on one side until bubbles form on the surface, then flip over and cook for another one to two more minutes.
5. Serve warm pancakes topped with your favorite toppings such as fresh berries, honey, maple syrup, and yogurt or nut butter.

**Nutrition (per serving):**

Calories: 300 kcal Protein: 10 g Carbohydrates: 45 g Fiber: 6 g Healthy Fats: 7 g

# 22. Breakfast Bake



## Ingredients

- 6 large eggs
- 1 cup of milk
- 2 cups of whole-grain bread, cubed
- 1 cup of cooked and crumbled turkey sausage or lean ham (optional)
- 1 cup of bell peppers, diced
- 1 cup of spinach, chopped
- 1/2 cup of onions, diced
- 1/2 cup of low-fat cheese, shredded (like cheddar or mozzarella)
- Salt and pepper, to taste
- Optional herbs: parsley, chives, or thyme

## Instructions

1. Preheat your oven to 375°F (190°C). Grease a baking pan with a bit of olive oil or cooking spray.
2. Evenly spread cubed bread in the baking pan.
3. Cooked sausage or ham (if preferred), diced bell peppers, chopped spinach and onions are layered over the bread.
4. Whisk together eggs, milk, salt and pepper in a bowl. After that, pour this mixture over the layer of bread and vegetables in the baking pan.
5. Sprinkle shredded cheese on top. Add any optional herbs for additional flavor.
6. Place in a preheated oven for 35 minutes until the eggs are set up and the top turns golden brown.
7. Allow breakfast bake to cool briefly before cutting into pieces and serving.

**Nutrition (per serving):**

Calories: 400 kcal Protein: 30 g Carbohydrates: 35 g Fiber: 6 g Healthy Fats: 20 g

# 23. Pumpkin Pancakes

**Prep Time: 10 minutes Cook Time: 15 minutes Servings: 3**

## Ingredients

- 1 cup of whole wheat flour
- 1/2 cup of pureed pumpkin
- 1 cup of milk
- 2 tbsp maple syrup or honey
- 1 large egg
- 2 tbsp melted butter or coconut oil
- 1 tsp baking powder
- 1/2 tsp baking soda
- 1/2 tsp ground cinnamon
- 1/4 tsp ground nutmeg
- 1/4 tsp ground ginger
- Pinch of salt
- Cooking spray or additional butter for the pan
- Optional toppings: extra maple syrup, chopped nuts, or fresh fruit

## Instructions

1. Combine flour, baking soda, baking powder, nutmeg, ginger, cinnamon and salt in a large bowl; whisk it together.
2. Mix pumpkin puree, melted butter, milk, maple syrup, and egg in another bowl.
3. Pour wet ingredients into dry ingredients and stir to combine. Avoid overmixing.
4. Heat a nonstick skillet or griddle over medium heat; spread with cooking spray or butter. Pour about 1/4 cup of batter for each pancake. Cook until bubbles appear on the surface, then flip the golden brown on the other side.
5. Serve the pancakes warm with your favorite toppings.

**Nutrition (per serving)**

Calories: 300 kcal Protein: 10 g Carbohydrates: 45 g Fiber: 7 g Healthy Fats: 12 g

# 24. Asparagus and Swiss cheese Frittata

**Prep Time: 10 minutes Cook Time: 20 minutes Servings: 2**

## Ingredients

- 6 large eggs
- 1/2 cup of Swiss cheese, shredded
- 1 cup of asparagus, trimmed and cut into 1-inch pieces
- 1/4 cup of milk
- 1 small onion, diced
- 2 tbsp olive oil
- Salt and pepper, to taste
- Optional: herbs such as thyme or parsley for added flavor

## Instructions

1. Preheat your oven to 375°F (190°C).
2. Warm the olive oil in an oven-proof skillet on medium flame. Throw in onion and asparagus. Cook until vegetables are tender, about 5-7 minutes.
3. Combine eggs, milk, salt and pepper in a bowl with a wire whisk. Sprinkle Swiss cheese over it and stir.
4. Add the egg mixture to the sautéed onions and asparagus in the pan; mix gently to combine.
5. Cook over medium heat for about five minutes or until the edges are set.
6. Put the skillet in the oven. Bake for 10-15 minutes or until the top is golden brown and the frittata is firm to touch.
7. Remove from oven; let cool for a few minutes. May garnish with fresh herbs, then cut into slices and serve.

**Nutrition (per serving):**

Calories: 350 kcal Protein: 25 g Carbohydrates: 10 g Fiber: 2 g Healthy Fats: 25 g

# 25. Maple Pecan Banana Muffins

**Prep Time: 15 minutes Cook Time: 25 minutes Servings: 12 muffins**

## Ingredients

- 1 ¾ cups of whole wheat flour
- 1 tsp baking soda
- 1/2 tsp salt
- 1/3 cup of pure maple syrup
- 1/2 cup of unsweetened applesauce
- 2 eggs
- 3 ripe bananas, mashed
- 1/4 cup of milk (dairy or plant-based)
- 1 tsp vanilla extract
- 1/2 cup of pecans, chopped
- Optional: additional pecans for topping

## Instructions

1. Preheat your oven to 350°F (175°C). Line a muffin tin with paper liners or grease the cups.
2. Whisk together the flour, baking soda, and salt in a large bowl.
3. Mix the maple syrup, applesauce, eggs, mashed bananas, milk and vanilla extract in another bowl.
4. Add the wet ingredients to the dry ones while stirring until they are combined. Avoid overmixing. Then, add the chopped pecans.
5. Put batter in muffin cups until about 3/4 full. You may sprinkle some pecan pieces on the top of each muffin for decoration.
6. Bake for 20-25 minutes or until a toothpick inserted into a muffin comes out clean at its center.
7. Let them cool inside the pan for five minutes before transferring them onto a wire rack to become cold throughout.

**Nutrition (per muffin):**

Calories: 220 kcal Protein: 6 g Carbohydrates: 30 g Fiber: 4 g Healthy Fats: 7 g

# 26. Clean Protein Power Bars

**Prep Time: 15 minutes Cook Time: 0 minutes Servings: 8-10 bars**

## Ingredients

- 1 cup of rolled oats
- 1/2 cup of protein powder
- 1/2 cup of almond butter
- 1/4 cup of honey or maple syrup
- 1/4 cup of milk
- 1/4 cup of chopped nuts
- 1/4 cup of seeds
- Optional: 1/4 cup of dark chocolate chips or dried fruit

## Instructions

1. Mix rolled oats, protein powder, nuts and seeds in a big bowl. If you want, you can include chocolate chips or dried fruits at this point.
2. In another bowl, mix almond butter, honey and milk. Mix them until they become appropriately combined.
3. Pour the wet mixture into the dry ingredients bowl. Mix all of it very well to ensure the mixture sticks together.
4. Put parchment paper on a baking pan or tray. Then, press the mixture evenly into the pan while ensuring it is firm.
5. Place the pan in a refrigerator and cool for about 2 hours until its consistency becomes solid.
6. Cut into bars or squares once chilled.

**Nutrition (per bar):**

Calories: 250 kcal Protein: 15 g Carbohydrates: 25 g Fiber: 5 g Healthy Fats: 12 g

# 27. Egg and Cheese Muffins

**Prep Time: 10 minutes Cook Time: 20 minutes Servings: 6 muffins**

## Ingredients

- 6 large eggs
- 1/2 cup of shredded cheese
- 1/4 cup of milk
- 1/2 cup of diced vegetables
- Salt and pepper, to taste
- Cooking spray or olive oil for greasing
- Optional: cooked and crumbled bacon or turkey bacon, herbs

## Instructions

1. Preheat the oven to 350°F. Grease a six-cup of muffin tin with cooking spray or olive oil.
2. Beat the eggs in a large bowl. Stir in milk, salt, and pepper until everything is well-mixed.
3. Add shredded cheese and chopped vegetables to it. If desired, add cooked bacon and herbs.
4. Pour equal amounts of egg mixture into each muffin cup.
5. Bake for 20 minutes or until the muffins are set and golden on top in a preheated oven.
6. Cool the muffins down for several minutes before removing them from the tin. Serve warm.

**Nutrition (per muffin):**

Calories: 120 kcal Protein: 10 g Carbohydrates: 3 g Fiber: 1 g Healthy Fats: 8 g

# 28. Cherry Protein Porridge

**Prep Time: 5 minutes Cook Time: 10 minutes Servings: 1**

## Ingredients

- 1/2 cup of rolled oats
- 1 cup of water or milk
- 1 scoop protein powder
- 1/2 cup of fresh or frozen cherries, pitted and halved
- 1 tbsp chopped nuts
- Optional: sweetener of choice to taste
- Optional: a sprinkle of cinnamon or vanilla extract for extra flavor

## Instructions

1. Bring milk or water to the boil in a saucepan. Put in rolled oats and reduce heat to low heat. Stir occasionally and cook for 5 minutes until the oats become soft.
2. Remove the saucepan from heat when the oats are cooked. Mix well with protein powder after adding. Add small amounts of water or milk to make it thinner if the porridge is too thick.
3. You can warm cherries if frozen or thaw them before stirring them into the pudding.
4. Sweeteners like cinnamon sprinkles, a sweetener of choice, or a few drops of vanilla extract may be added as desired.
5. Place chopped nuts on top, then pour the mixture into a bowl.

**Nutrition (per serving):**

Calories: 350 kcal Protein: 25 g Carbohydrates: 45 g Fiber: 7 g Healthy Fats: 7 g

# 29. Chocolate Banana Protein Pancakes

**Prep Time: 10 minutes Cook Time: 10 minutes Servings: 2**

## Ingredients

- 1 medium ripe banana
- 2 large eggs
- 1 scoop of chocolate protein powder
- 1/4 cup of oat flour or almond flour
- 1 tbsp cocoa powder
- 1/2 tsp baking powder
- A pinch of salt
- Cooking spray or coconut oil for the pan
- Optional toppings: fresh banana slices, a drizzle of honey or maple syrup, Greek yogurt, or nut butter

## Instructions

1. Using a big bowl, crush the banana with a fork till it is creamy.
2. Crack the eggs into your bowl with mashed banana and mix well.
3. Mix in chocolate protein powder, oat or almond flour, cocoa powder, baking powder, and a pinch of salt until the batter is combined.
4. Place non-stick skillet on medium heat and lightly grease with cooking spray or coconut oil. Pour about ¼ cup of batter for each pancake. Cook for 2-3 minutes on one side, then bubbles appear. Flip and cook for another 1-2 minutes.
5. Serve pancakes hot with desired toppings like fresh banana slices and some honey Greek yogurt or nut butter drizzles.

**Nutrition (per serving):**

Calories: 320 kcal Protein: 25 g Carbohydrates: 35 g Fiber: 5 g Healthy Fats: 10 g

# 30. Homemade Scallion Hash Brown Cakes

**Prep Time: 15 minutes Cook Time: 15 minutes Servings: 4 cakes**

## Ingredients

- 2 large russet potatoes, peeled and grated
- 2 scallions, finely chopped
- 1 large egg, beaten
- 2 tbsp all-purpose flour
- Salt and pepper, to taste
- 2-3 tbsp olive oil for frying
- Optional: 1/4 tsp garlic powder or paprika for added flavor

## Instructions

1. Place the grated potatoes in a clean dish towel and squeeze them as much as possible. This is necessary for making crispy hash browns.
2. In a bowl, combine the drained grated potatoes, chopped green onions, beaten egg, flour, salt, pepper, garlic powder and paprika if using. Mix well.
3. Divide the mixture into 4 equal parts. Shape each part into a round, flat cake.
4. Put olive oil in a large skillet and heat it over medium heat. Put hash brown cakes on the pan and press with a spatula until they become flat. Cook for about 6 to 7 minutes per side or until golden brown.
5. After cooking, transfer the hash brown cakes to a paper towel-lined plate to drain any excess oil. Serve hot.

### Nutrition

Calories: 220 kcal Protein: 4 g Carbohydrates: 25 g Fiber: 2 g Healthy Fats: 10 g

## 1. Lentil Soup

**Prep Time: 10 minutes Cook Time: 45 minutes Servings: 4-6**

## Ingredients

- 1 cup of dried lentils (green, brown, or red)
- 1 large onion, diced
- 2 carrots, diced
- 2 celery stalks, diced
- 2 garlic cloves, minced
- 1 can diced tomatoes
- 6 cups of vegetable broth or water
- 1 tsp ground cumin
- 1/2 tsp dried thyme
- Salt and pepper, to taste
- 2 tbsp olive oil
- Optional: 1 bay leaf, a squeeze of lemon juice, chopped fresh parsley for garnish.

## Instructions

1. Heat the olive oil in a large pot over medium heat. Add the onion, carrots, celery and garlic to the pot, then you can sauté for about 5 minutes until the vegetables get softened.
2. Drain lentils before adding them to the pot. Lentils should be supplemented with diced tomatoes, vegetable broth, cumin, thyme and bay leaf (if desired). Add salt and pepper to taste.
3. Boil soup and reduce its heat before allowing it to simmer for approximately 35-40 minutes or until the lentils become tender.
4. Keep aside bay leaf and adjust seasoning as required. One can lightly blend several portions of the soup with an immersion blender, giving it a little thicker texture.
5. Pour soup into bowls. One may garnish with chopped parsley or squeeze lemon on it.

**Nutrition (per serving):**

Calories: 200 kcal Protein: 15 g Carbohydrates: 35 g Fiber: 10 g Healthy Fats: 5 g

# 2. Vegetable Soup

**Prep Time: 15 minutes Cook Time: 30 minutes Servings: 4-6**

## Ingredients

- 2 tbsp olive oil
- 1 large onion, diced
- 2 carrots, peeled and diced
- 2 celery stalks, diced
- 2 garlic cloves, minced
- 1 zucchini, diced
- 1 bell pepper, diced
- 1 cup of green beans, trimmed and cut into 1-inch pieces
- 1 can diced tomatoes (with juice)
- 6 cups of vegetable broth
- 1 tsp dried basil
- 1 tsp dried oregano
- Salt and pepper, to taste
- Optional: 1 cup of spinach or kale, chopped

## Instructions

1. Let a lot of heat in a large pot with olive oil. Put onion, carrot and celery; fry for about five minutes until tender. Garlic can also be added and cooked for one more minute.
2. Incorporate zucchini into the mixture after stirring bell pepper and green beans. Cook it for 3-4 minutes.
3. Add vegetable broth as well as diced tomatoes (with their juice). Season it with basil, oregano, salt and pepper.
4. Afterwards, simmer the soup uncovered for 20 minutes or until vegetables are soft over low heat, having previously brought it to a boil at the first point.
5. To that effect, add spinach or kale while cooking towards the end, then let them wilt a bit in the process.
6. To ensure everything is okay, taste and correct seasoning before serving hot.

**Nutrition (per serving):**

Calories: 150 kcal Protein: 3 g Carbohydrates: 18 g Fiber: 5 g Healthy Fats: 5 g

# 3. Lentil Stew

**Prep Time: 15 minutes Cook Time: 45 minutes Servings: 4**

## Ingredients

- 1 cup of dried lentils
- 1 large onion, chopped
- 2 carrots, diced
- 2 celery stalks, diced
- 3 garlic cloves, minced
- 1 can (14.5 oz) diced tomatoes
- 6 cups of vegetable or chicken broth
- 2 tsp ground cumin
- 1 tsp paprika
- 1/2 tsp dried thyme
- Salt and pepper, to taste
- 2 tbsp olive oil
- Optional: 1 bay leaf, 1 cup of chopped spinach or kale, lemon juice, and fresh parsley for garnish

## Instructions

1. Heat the olive oil in a large pot on a medium head. Onion, carrots and celery should be added. The vegetables should be sautéed until they soften, which will take approximately five minutes. Sauté garlic for one minute.
2. Wash lentils; place them in the pot along with diced tomatoes, vegetable or chicken broth, cumin, paprika, thyme and bay leaf (if used). Adjust salt and pepper according to taste.
3. The mixture is then allowed to boil before reducing the heat, simmering and covering it for 35-40 minutes till the lentils are tender.
4. If you have spinach or kale, mix it in only during the last few minutes of cooking and let it wilt.
5. The bay leaf can be removed if needed. Seasoning can be adjusted as required; a squeeze of lemon juice may be added for zesting.
6. Put stew into bowls using a spoon. Optionally garnish with fresh parsley or leave plain.

**Nutrition (per serving):**

Calories: 250 kcal Protein: 15 g Carbohydrates: 35 g Fiber: 12 g Healthy Fats: 5 g

# 4. Artichoke and Olive Pasta

**Prep Time: 10 minutes Cook Time: 20 minutes Servings: 4**

## Ingredients

- 8 oz whole grain or lentil pasta
- 1 can (14 oz) artichoke hearts, drained and quartered
- 1/2 cup of Kalamata olives, pitted and sliced
- 2 garlic cloves, minced
- 1/2 cup of cherry tomatoes, halved
- 1/4 cup of extra virgin olive oil
- 1/4 cup of grated Parmesan cheese
- Salt and pepper, to taste
- 2 tbsp fresh basil, chopped
- 1 tbsp lemon juice
- Optional: Red pepper flakes for a spicy kick

## Instructions

1. Following instructions on the package, cook the pasta in boiling salted water until it is al dente. Drain and place aside, leaving 1/2 cup of pasta water.
2. Add olive oil and heat over medium flame in a skillet that is big enough. Fry garlic for 60 seconds. Stir in artichoke hearts and cook for four minutes.
3. Stir Kalamata olives and cherry tomatoes into the mixture. Cook for three minutes again.
4. Pour the cooked pasta into the pan while stirring well to combine with vegetables. To make it juicy, a little of the reserved pasta water may be added if it feels too dry.
5. Season with lemon juice, fresh basil and grated Parmesan cheese. Add salt, pepper and red pepper flakes (optional).
6. Serve the hot pasta topped with extra basil or Parmesan cheese, depending on your taste buds.

**Nutrition (per serving):**

Calories: 380 kcal Protein: 12 g Carbohydrates: 45 g Fiber: 9 g Healthy Fats: 18 g

# 5. Vegetable Pasta

**Prep Time: 15 minutes Cook Time: 20 minutes Servings: 4**

## Ingredients

- 8 oz whole wheat or legume-based pasta
- 2 tbsp olive oil
- 1 zucchini, sliced
- 1 bell pepper, diced
- 1 small eggplant, cubed
- 1/2 cup of cherry tomatoes, halved
- 2 cloves garlic, minced
- 1/2 cup of onion, chopped
- 1/4 cup of fresh basil, chopped
- 1/4 cup of grated Parmesan cheese (optional)
- Salt and pepper, to taste
- Optional: red pepper flakes, for heat

## Instructions

1. Get the pasta cooked until al dente according to the instructions provided on its pack. Drain and keep aside.
2. Put olive oil over heat in a large frying pan/frying skillet. Add onion and garlic, sautéing until it smells delicious. Add zucchini, bell pepper and eggplant. Cook for about 7-10 minutes until vegetables become tender.
3. Mix in cherry tomatoes and cook for another two to three minutes.
4. Combine cooked pasta with vegetables in the skillet. Toss up gently to combine them well. Heat through.
5. Put fresh basil, salt, pepper, and red pepper flakes in this bowl. Now mix well.
6. If you want to top your bowl of pasta with grated parmesan cheese, then go ahead.

**Nutrition (per serving):**

Calories: 320 kcal Protein: 12 g Carbohydrates: 55 g Fiber: 10 g Healthy Fats: 10 g

# 6. High-Protein Spaghetti



## Ingredients

- 8 oz high-protein spaghetti
- 1 pound lean ground turkey or chicken
- 1 jar marinara sauce
- 1 onion, diced
- 2 garlic cloves, minced
- 2 tbsp olive oil
- Salt and pepper, to taste
- Optional: red pepper flakes, fresh herbs, grated Parmesan cheese

## Instructions

1. Boil the spaghetti with high protein according to the salt-sprinkled water al dente procedure as per the instructions on the package. Then, drain and set aside.
2. Bring 1 tablespoon of olive oil to boiling point under medium heat in a large skillet. After which, add ground turkey or chicken and cook until well browned and fully cooked through seasoning with salt and pepper. Remove them from the skillet, then set aside.
3. Add the remaining olive oil to the same skillet. Add onion diced in small pieces until it becomes clear, like cellophane paper, then pour in minced garlic and continue frying for another minute.
4. Return the beef to the skillet after cooking it. Mix marinara sauce well with it; then add some red pepper flakes to give it a sweet taste if you wish.
5. Turn down the heat and let it simmer for about ten minutes to combine all flavors properly.
6. Put the cooked pasta into the sauce while stirring it occasionally to cover all parts of the pasta evenly.
7. When ready, serve the plate with hot spaghetti garnished with desired fresh spices and grated Parmesan cheese.

**Nutrition (per serving)**

Calories: 380 kcal Protein: 30 g Carbohydrates: 42 g Fiber: 7 g Healthy Fats: 10 g

# 7. Muscle Lentil Soup

**Prep Time: 10 minutes Cook Time: 45 minutes Servings: 4-6**

## Ingredients

- 1 cup of dried green or brown lentils
- 1 large onion, chopped
- 2 carrots, diced
- 2 celery stalks, diced
- 3 garlic cloves, minced
- 1 can diced tomatoes with juice
- 6 cups of chicken or vegetable broth
- 2 tsp ground cumin
- 1 tsp smoked paprika
- 1/2 tsp dried thyme
- Salt and pepper, to taste
- 2 tbsp olive oil
- Optional: 1 bay leaf, 2 cups of chopped spinach or kale, and lemon wedges for serving

## Instructions

1. Place the olive oil in a large pot and heat over medium-high temperature. After that, sauté garlic, onions, celery, and carrots until they get soft.
2. Wash lentils and transfer them into the pot. Bring some diced tomatoes, broth, cumin seeds or powder, paprika, thyme leaves and bay leaf. You should also sprinkle salt and pepper onto the soup.
3. Boil the soup, then lower the flame to simmer it for about 35-40 minutes, covered until the lentils become soft.
4. If you are using spinach or kale, add them during the last stages of cooking so that they fade away quickly.
5. Add spices if necessary. Remove the bay leaf from the pot. Lemon wedges may be served with this hot soup.

**Nutrition (per serving):**

Calories: 270 kcal Protein: 20 g Carbohydrates: 35 g Fiber: 12 g Healthy Fats: 7 g

# 8. Mediterranean Shrimp Penne

**Prep Time: 15 minutes Cook Time: 20 minutes Servings: 4**

## Ingredients

- 8 oz whole grain or lentil penne pasta
- 1 pound shrimp, peeled and deveined
- 2 tbsp olive oil
- 1 onion, diced
- 3 garlic cloves, minced
- 1 can diced tomatoes, drained
- 1/2 cup of Kalamata olives, pitted and sliced
- 1/4 cup of capers
- 1/2 cup of feta cheese, crumbled
- 1/4 cup of fresh basil, chopped
- Salt and pepper, to taste
- Optional: Red pepper flakes, lemon zest, or a splash of white wine

## Instructions

1. Boil the penne in salted water according to package instructions. Drain and set aside.
2. Heat 1 tablespoon olive oil over medium heat in a large skillet until hot. Salt and pepper the shrimp, then cook until they are pink, for about 2-3 minutes per side. Remove them from the skillet and set aside.
3. In the same skillet, add the rest of the olive oil. Sauté onions and garlic till translucent.
4. Throw in diced tomatoes, Kalamata olives, and capers. Cook for approximately five minutes; if desired, enhance it with white wine or lemon zest.
5. Introduce penne that has been cooked into this mixture together with shrimp. Toss well to combine and warm through.
6. Take away from the oven. Mix feta cheese and fresh basil leaves while seasoning with salt, pepper or red pepper flakes.
7. Serve hot pasta topped with more basil or cheese if desired.

**Nutrition (per serving):**

Calories: 420 kcal Protein: 28 g Carbohydrates: 45 g Fiber: 7 g Healthy Fats: 18 g

# 9. Whole Wheat Pasta with Marinara Sauce

**Prep Time: 5 minutes Cook Time: 20 minutes Servings: 4**

## Ingredients

- 8 oz whole wheat spaghetti or pasta of your choice
- 2 cups of marinara sauce
- 2 tbsp olive oil
- 2 garlic cloves, minced
- 1/2 tsp dried basil
- 1/2 tsp dried oregano
- Salt and pepper, to taste
- Optional: red pepper flakes, grated Parmesan cheese, fresh basil for garnish

## Instructions

1. Cook the whole wheat pasta in a large pot of boiling, salted water until tender, as directed on the package. Set aside after draining.
2. Heat olive oil in a saucepan over medium heat while the pasta is cooking. Put minced garlic into it and stir for around one minute till the aroma rises. Be cautious not to make it burn.
3. Add the marinara sauce to the pan. Add dried basil, oregano, salt and black pepper. If you want some heat, throw in some red chili flakes. Cook uncovered for 10 minutes, stirring occasionally.
4. Once cooked, add pasta to the marinara saucepan. Mix properly so the sauce spreads uniformly on each pasta strand.
5. If desired, pasta should be served hot with grated Parmesan cheese and fresh basil leaves.

**Nutrition (per serving):**

Calories: 320 kcal Protein: 10 g Carbohydrates: 60 g Fiber: 10 g Healthy Fats: 8 g

# 10. Quick Ramen with Shredded Chicken

**Prep Time: 10 minutes Cook Time: 20 minutes Servings: 2**

## Ingredients

- 2 packs of instant ramen noodles
- 1 cup of cooked chicken, shredded
- 4 cups of chicken broth (low-sodium)
- 1 carrot, thinly sliced
- 1 cup of baby spinach or bok choy
- 2 green onions, chopped
- 1 tbsp soy sauce (low-sodium)
- 1 tsp sesame oil
- 1 garlic clove, minced
- Optional: boiled egg, sliced mushrooms, sesame seeds, chili flakes

## Instructions

1. Boil the chicken broth in a saucepan. Put in minced garlic and soy sauce.
2. Put the ramen noodles into the broth. Cook for 2 -3 minutes as directed on the pack.
3. Add Carrot slices, spinach, and shredded chicken to this. Cook for 2-3 more minutes until the vegetables are tender and the chicken is warmed.
4. Mix it with sesame oil. Readjust the taste if necessary by pouring more soy sauce or chili flakes to make it hotter.
5. Share the soup with ramen in two bowls. Add chopped green onions for garnish or other optional toppings, including boiled egg, mushrooms, sesame seeds, etc.

**Nutrition (per serving):**

Calories: 350 kcal Protein: 28 g Carbohydrates: 42 g Fiber: 4 g Healthy Fats: 10 g

# 11. Traditional Shrimp Scampi

**Prep Time: 10 minutes Cook Time: 10 minutes Servings: 4**

## Ingredients

- 1 pound large shrimp, peeled and deveined
- 8 oz spaghetti or linguine
- 4 tbsp unsalted butter
- 4 tbsp olive oil
- 4 garlic cloves, minced
- 1/2 cup of dry white wine
- Juice of 1 lemon
- Zest of 1 lemon
- 1/4 cup of parsley, finely chopped
- Salt and pepper, to taste
- Red pepper flakes (optional, for heat)
- Grated Parmesan cheese (optional for serving)

## Instructions

1. The pasta is cooked according to the package in salted water until al dente. Drain it and leave it aside while keeping 1/2 cup of pasta water.
2. Put 2 tablespoon of olive oil into a large skillet, then put the heat on medium-high. Salt and pepper your shrimp. Cook them for about one to two minutes on each side or until they become pinkish in color and opaque. Remove the shrimp from the pan.
3. In the same skillet, reduce heat to medium-low. Add remaining olive oil with butter. Once melted, add minced garlic while being cautious not to burn it, and then cook for a minute. Finally, pour in white wine (or chicken broth) with lemon juice; let the mixture simmer for 2-3 minutes to reduce it slightly.
4. Return shrimp to skillet, then add cooked pasta, grated lemon zest, and chopped parsley. Mix everything by tossing before adding reserved pasta water if it feels too dry.
5. You can garnish with more parsley, red pepper flakes, and grated Parmesan cheese when serving immediately.

**Nutrition (per serving):**

Calories: 450 kcal Protein: 30 g Carbohydrates: 45 g Fiber: 3 g Healthy Fats: 20 g

# 12. Sweet Potato & Green Pea Soup

**Prep Time: 10 minutes Cook Time: 30 minutes Servings: 4**

## Ingredients

- 2 large sweet potatoes, peeled and diced
- 1 cup of green peas (fresh or frozen)
- 1 onion, diced
- 2 garlic cloves, minced
- 4 cups of vegetable broth
- 1 tsp ground cumin
- 1/2 tsp paprika
- Salt and pepper, to taste
- 2 tbsp olive oil

Optional: a dash of nutmeg, coconut milk for creaminess, fresh herbs like parsley or cilantro for garnish

## Instructions

1. Heat olive oil using a large pot over medium heat. Add the chopped onion and crushed garlic, cooking to this step until it turns brown.
2. For almost ten minutes, stir-fry the sweet potatoes that are diced.
3. Scatter cumin powder, paprika, salt, and pepper into the mix, then pour vegetable stock into it before boiling.
4. Cook for 20 minutes more under low heat or until sweet potatoes are cooked.
5. In addition, put peas in the same pot and boil them for five minutes further.
6. Use an immersion blender to blend the soup until smooth. Instead of using an immersion blender if you don't have one, you can puree soup carefully with a regular blender.
7. Coconut milk may be added to make it creamier in texture. Adjust seasoning accordingly.
8. When served hot, garnish the soup with fresh herbs or sprinkle some nutmeg powder on top; alternatively, adding a drizzle of olive oil will also do.

**Nutrition (per serving)**

Calories: 220 kcal Protein: 5 g Carbohydrates: 35 g Fiber: 7 g Healthy Fats: 8 g

# 13. Bell Pasta with Kidney Beans

**Prep Time: 10 minutes Cook Time: 20 minutes Servings: 4**

## Ingredients

- 8 oz whole wheat pasta
- 1 can (15 oz) kidney beans, drained and rinsed
- 1 red bell pepper, diced
- 1 green bell pepper, diced
- 1 onion, diced
- 2 garlic cloves, minced
- 1 can (14.5 oz) diced tomatoes
- 2 tbsp olive oil
- 1 tsp dried oregano
- 1 tsp dried basil
- Salt and pepper, to taste

Optional: red pepper flakes, grated Parmesan cheese, fresh parsley or basil for garnish

## Instructions

1. Follow the directions on the package to cook the whole-wheat pasta until it is al dente. After that, drain and set aside.
2. Heat 1 tablespoon of olive oil over medium heat in a big frying pan. Add chopped onion, bell pepper and garlic that you have ground so that they become tender for about 5-7 minutes.
3. Put in kidney beans and canned tomatoes (with their juice). Also, season with some oregano, basil, salt and pepper. If you want it hot, then you can always add red pepper flakes.
4. Stir occasionally and allow simmering for about 10 minutes.
5. Finally, put cooked pasta into the skillet with vegetable mixture and toss gently to mix them well.
6. If desired, serve with parmesan cheese or fresh parsley or basil on top when serving hot pasta.

**Nutrition (per serving)**

Calories: 370 kcal Protein: 180 g Carbohydrates: 60 g Fiber: 10 g Healthy Fats: 8 g

# 14. Farfalle with Chicken and Pesto

**Prep Time: 15 minutes Cook Time: 20 minutes Servings: 4**

## Ingredients

- 8 oz farfalle (bow-tie) pasta
- 2 boneless, skinless chicken breasts
- 1/2 cup of basil pesto
- 2 tbsp olive oil
- 2 garlic cloves, minced
- 1/2 cup of cherry tomatoes, halved
- 1/4 cup of grated Parmesan cheese
- Salt and pepper, to taste

Optional: red pepper flakes, additional basil leaves for garnish

## Instructions

1. Cook the farfalle until it is al dente in a large pot of boiling, salted water according to package directions. Then, drain and put aside.
2. Put some salt and pepper on the chicken pieces. Cook them in a big frying pan and heat olive oil over medium heat. Brown and cook it for roughly six to eight minutes, then mix garlic at the last minute.
3. Reduce the temperature to low. Add basil pesto with cooked farfalle onto a skillet containing chicken. Toss pesto until it is evenly coated with pasta.
4. Stir in cherry tomatoes and cook for another 2 minutes until they are slightly softened.
5. Sprinkle grated Parmesan cheese over hot pasta; serve with red pepper flakes sprinkled on top if desired; add more fresh basil as garnish if desired.

**Nutrition (per serving):**

Calories: 450 kcal Protein: 25 g Carbohydrates: 50 g Fiber: 4 g Healthy Fats: 20 g

# 15. Spicy Buffalo Macaroni and Cheese

**Prep Time: 15 minutes Cook Time: 20 minutes Servings: 4**

## Ingredients

- 8 oz elbow macaroni
- 2 cups of shredded cheddar cheese
- 1/2 cup of cream cheese
- 1/2 cup of buffalo sauce
- 1/2 cup of milk (dairy or plant-based)
- 2 tbsp unsalted butter
- 1/2 cup of breadcrumbs
- 2 tbsp olive oil
- 1/4 cup of blue cheese crumbles (optional)
- 2 green onions, chopped
- Salt and pepper, to taste

Optional: 1/2 cup of cooked and shredded chicken for added protein

## Instructions

1. Macaroni should be cooked as quickly as possible as per the directions provided in the package. It is then drained and set aside.
2. Next, melt butter in a saucepan over medium heat. Cream cheese and milk are added, stirring until smooth. Gradually whisk in the cheddar cheese while stirring continuously until it has completely melted and has become creamy.
3. Buffalo sauce is stirred into the mixture and then seasoned with salt and pepper to taste; this is where you add shredded chicken.
4. The cheese sauce prepared earlier is now mixed with macaroni that has already been cooked. The aim here is to have every strand of macaroni covered by the sauce.
5. In a little bowl, combine breadcrumbs with olive oil.
6. Preheat oven to 375°F (190°C). The Macaroni mixture should be transferred to the baking pan. Top with breadcrumb mixture and sprinkle evenly over the casserole pan. Bake for 10-15 minutes or until top is golden brown and crisp.
7. Lastly, garnish with blue cheese crumbles and chopped green onions.
8. Serve spicy buffalo macaroni cheese hot.

**Nutrition (per serving):**

Calories: 550 kcal Protein: 25 g Carbohydrates: 55 g Fiber: 2 g Healthy Fats: 30 g

# 16. Cream of Broccoli Soup

**Prep Time: 10 minutes Cook Time: 20 minutes Servings: 4**

## Ingredients

- 4 cups of broccoli florets
- 1 onion, chopped
- 2 garlic cloves, minced
- 3 cups of vegetable or chicken broth
- 1 cup of milk
- 2 tbsp butter or olive oil
- 2 tbsp all-purpose flour
- Salt and pepper, to taste

Optional: 1/2 cup of grated cheddar cheese, nutmeg, and a dollop of cream for serving

## Instructions

1. In a large pot, melt the butter or heat the olive oil over medium flame. Sauté until the onion becomes translucent.
2. Cook for 3-4 minutes in the pot by stirring occasionally after adding broccoli florets.
3. Put flour on broccoli and stir; cook for 1 minute more.
4. After putting in the broth, pour and mix while boiling. Then simmer it until the broccoli is tender, about 10 minutes.
5. Puree soup using an immersion blender to make it smooth in the pot. Alternatively, you can blend the soup until smooth in batches with a regular blender.
6. Put back soup into the pot (if you are using a blender). Heat through while mixing in milk, but don't boil. Add, if necessary, salt and pepper. Lastly, sprinkle grated cheddar cheese if desired, then melt when stirred.
7. Serve hot with some sprinkles of nutmeg and top up with some cream, as needed.

**Nutrition (per serving)**

Calories: 200 kcal Protein: 8 g Carbohydrates: 20 g Fiber: 5 g Healthy Fats: 10 g

# CHAPTER 3: BEEF, PORK, AND POULTRY

## 1. Beef Shish Kebabs

**Prep Time: 30 minutes Cook Time: 10-15 minutes Servings: 4**

### Ingredients

- 1 ½ pounds beef sirloin,
- 1 bell pepper (any color)
- 1 large onion
- 1 zucchini
- 1 cup of cherry tomatoes
- 1/4 cup of olive oil
- 3 tbsp soy sauce (low-sodium)
- 2 tbsp lemon juice
- 2 garlic cloves, minced
- 1 tsp dried oregano
- 1/2 tsp ground black pepper
- Salt to taste
- Wooden or metal skewers

### Instructions

1. Take a mixing bowl and combine olive oil, soy sauce, lemon juice, chopped garlic, oregano, black pepper and salt by whisking them with a fork. Put in beef cubes and mix them well. Cover the mixture with foil or a lid and refrigerate for at least two hours or, better still, overnight.
2. Heat an outdoor grill to medium-high heat. Those using wooden kabob skewers should be soaked in water for half an hour to avoid burning.
3. Marinate bell peppers, onions, zucchini and cherry tomatoes in beef. After marinating these ingredients for quite some time, it is high time you thread them on a skewer alternately with meat.
4. Place kebabs on a preheated grill. Occasionally, turn them for 10-15 minutes until the desired degree of doneness of beef is reached.
5. Remove the skewers from the grill and leave aside for some time before serving.

**Nutrition (per serving):**

Calories: 450 kcal Protein: 40 g Carbohydrates: 10 g Fiber: 2 g Healthy Fats: 20 g

# 2. Classic Steak

**Prep Time: 5 minutes Cook Time: 10 minutes Servings: 2**

## Ingredients

- 2 steaks
- 2 tbsp olive oil or vegetable oil
- Salt and freshly ground black pepper to taste

Optional: 2 garlic cloves, 2 sprigs of fresh thyme or rosemary, 2 tbsp butter

## Instructions

1. To reach room temperature, remove the steaks from the refrigerator at least 30 minutes before cooking. This way, even heating will be ensured.
2. A heavy skillet (preferably cast iron) should be heated over high heat. Add oil to the pan and heat until it shimmers but does not smoke.
3. Salt and pepper are heavily on both sides of the steaks.
4. Place in a hot skillet. For medium-rare, cook about 4-6 minutes on each side or longer for medium to well-done. If you are using it, when you flip over the steak, add butter, garlic, and herbs and baste it with melted butter.
5. Take it out of the pan and rest on a cutting board or plate for about 5 minutes before slicing, enabling juices to be spread throughout the meat again.

**Nutrition (per serving):**

Calories: 450 kcal Protein: 45 g Carbohydrates: 0 g Fiber: 0 g Healthy Fats: 35 g

# 3. Lemon-Herb Grilled Chicken Salad

**Prep Time: 20 minutes Cook Time: 10-15 minutes Servings: 4**

## Ingredients

For the Chicken:

- 4 boneless, skinless chicken breasts
- 2 tbsp olive oil
- Juice and zest of 1 lemon
- 2 garlic cloves, minced
- 1 tsp dried oregano
- 1 tsp dried basil
- Salt and pepper, to taste

For the Salad:

- 8 cups of mixed salad greens
- 1 cucumber, sliced
- 1 cup of cherry tomatoes, halved
- 1/2 red onion, thinly sliced
- 1/4 cup of Kalamata olives, pitted and halved
- 1/4 cup of feta cheese, crumbled
- Optional: additional lemon wedges for serving

For the Dressing:

- 1/4 cup of olive oil
- 2 tbsp lemon juice
- 1 tsp Dijon mustard
- 1 garlic clove, minced
- Salt and pepper, to taste

## Instructions

1. Whisk olive oil, lemon juice, zest, minced garlic, oregano, basil, salt, and pepper in a bowl. Marinate the chicken breasts in this mixture, ensuring they are fully covered. Keep refrigerated for at least 30 minutes or longer.
2. Preheat the grill to medium-high heat. Grill the chicken for about 5 to 7 minutes per side until it is cooked thoroughly and reaches an internal temperature of 165 degrees Fahrenheit (75 degrees Celsius). Let it sit for a while, then cut into pieces.

3. Whisk together olive oil, lemon juice, Dijon mustard, minced garlic, salt and pepper in a small bowl to make the dressing.
4. Combine mixed greens, cucumber, cherry tomatoes, red onion, and olives in a large mixing bowl. Drizzle over salad, then toss to coat it with the dressing.
5. Serve salad on plates. Sprinkle slices of grilled chicken on top, followed by crumbled feta cheese. Served as one wishes with more wedges of lemons.

**Nutrition (per serving):**

Calories: 350 kcal Protein: 30 g Carbohydrates: 15 g Fiber: 3 g Healthy Fats: 20 g

# 4. Pork Loin with Baked Apples

**Prep Time: 15 minutes Cook Time: 50 minutes Servings: 4**

## Ingredients

- 1 pork loin
- 4 apples, cored and sliced
- 2 tbsp olive oil
- 2 tbsp honey or maple syrup
- 2 tbsp Dijon mustard
- 1 tsp dried thyme
- 1 tsp dried rosemary
- Salt and pepper, to taste
- Optional: fresh herbs for garnish

## Instructions

1. Preheat your oven to 375°F (190°C).
2. Olive oil, pepper and salt are used to rub the pork loin. Rosemary and dried thyme should be sprinkled over.
3. In a bowl, slice the apple and mix it with maple syrup or honey.
4. Put the pork loin in a roasting pan. Arrange slices of apple around it. Spread some Dijon mustard on top of it.
5. Roast it in an oven preheated up to 63°C for approximately forty-five to sixty minutes until you get an inside temperature of 145°F. Baste occasionally using pan juices.
6. Let the pork loin settle for ten minutes when taken out of the oven. After that, you can slice it and serve it with baked apples. You may sprinkle fresh herbs as garnish if needed.

Calories: 450 kcal Protein: 45 g Carbohydrates: 25 g Fiber: 4 g Healthy Fats: 25 g

# 5. Japanese Steak Curry

**Prep Time: 15 minutes Cook Time: 45 minutes Servings: 4**

## Ingredients

- 1 pound beef steak, cut into cubes
- 4 cups of beef broth
- 1 large onion, sliced
- 2 carrots, peeled and sliced
- 2 potatoes, peeled and cubed
- 1 apple, peeled and grated
- 3 tbsp vegetable oil
- 3 tbsp Japanese curry powder
- 1 garlic clove, minced
- 1 tbsp ginger, grated
- 2 tbsp soy sauce
- 1 tbsp Worcestershire sauce
- 1 bay leaf
- Salt and pepper, to taste
- Cooked rice for serving

## Instructions

1. A large pot is heated over medium-high heat with vegetable oil of one tbsp. The steak cubes should be seasoned with pepper and salt. This continues until the beef is browned, keeping in mind not to crowd the pot. Steaks are then left aside.
2. In this same pan, add tablespoon of oil. These should be sautéed for about 5 minutes.
3. The minced garlic and grated ginger will also be included. Cook for another minute till fragrant.
4. Steak must be returned to the pot while beef broth, curry powder, grated apple, soy sauce, Worcestershire sauce, and bay leaf must be added. Stir well to combine.
5. Let the mixture boil before simmering at low heat for 30 minutes or until the meat becomes tender and the potatoes get cooked through.
6. Remove bay leaves; taste and adjust seasoning using pepper and salt when necessary.
7. Serve the Japanese Steak Curry over cooked rice.

# 6. Low-Fat Chicken Bacon Ranch Sandwich

**Prep Time: 15 minutes Cook Time: 15 minutes Servings: 4**

## Ingredients

- 4 boneless, skinless chicken breasts
- 8 slices of turkey bacon
- 4 whole wheat sandwich buns
- 1/2 cup of low-fat ranch dressing
- 1 tomato, sliced
- 4 lettuce leaves
- 1 avocado, sliced (optional)
- Salt and pepper, to taste
- Cooking spray or a small amount of olive oil

## Instructions

1. Just season the chicken breasts with salt and pepper. Heat a grill pan or skillet to medium, lightly spritz it with cooking spray, or sprinkle some olive oil. You should grill the chicken for 6-7 minutes on each side until it is thoroughly cooked and the internal temperature reaches its maximum of not less than 165°F (75°C). Take off the heat, then allow it a few minutes.
2. Meanwhile, cook turkey bacon in the same frying pan until very crispy, approximately three minutes on either side.
3. If desired, you could toast whole wheat buns. Every bun must be applied with a light layer of low-fat ranch dressing. Add a grilled chicken breast, two slices of turkey bacon, lettuce leaves, tomato slices, and avocado pieces, if using any.
4. Then, close these sandwiches using the upper halves of the buns and serve them immediately.

**Nutrition (per serving):**

Calories: 350 kcal Protein: 35 g Carbohydrates: 30 g Fiber: 5 g Healthy Fats: 8 g

# 7. Macro Roast Beef

**Prep Time: 15 minutes Cook Time: 60 minutes Servings: 4**

## Ingredients

- 2 pounds beef sirloin tip roast
- 2 tbsp olive oil
- 2 garlic cloves, minced
- 1 tsp dried rosemary
- 1 tsp dried thyme
- Salt and pepper, to taste
- Optional: vegetables for roasting, cut into chunks

## Instructions

1. Preheat your oven to 375°F (190°C).
2. Oil the beef using olive oil. Sprinkle garlic, rosemary, thyme, salt and pepper on opposite sides of the meat.
3. Put it in a roasting pan, and if you incorporate vegetables, scatter them around it. Cook in an oven for about 60-90 minutes or until your desired level of doneness is achieved (145°F for medium-rare, 160°F for medium).
4. When the meat is ready, take it out of the oven and allow it to sit for 10-15 minutes before carving. This helps in redistributing the juices.
5. Finally, cut into slices and serve with roasted vegetables.

**Nutrition (per serving):**

Calories: 350 kcal Protein: 45 g Carbohydrates: 5 g Fiber: 1 g Healthy Fats: 20 g

# 8. Chicken Chili

**Prep Time: 15 minutes Cook Time: 1 hour Servings: 6**

## Ingredients

- 2 tbsp olive oil
- 1 large onion, diced
- 2 garlic cloves, minced
- 1 bell pepper (any color), diced
- 1 jalapeño, seeded and minced
- 1 ½ pounds boneless, skinless chicken breasts cut into bite-sized pieces
- 2 cans white beans, drained and rinsed
- 1 can diced tomatoes
- 4 cups of chicken broth
- 1 tbsp chili powder
- 1 tsp ground cumin
- 1 tsp dried oregano
- Salt and pepper, to taste

Optional toppings: chopped cilantro, shredded cheese, sour cream, avocado slices

## Instructions

1. Heat the olive oil in a large pot on medium heat. Throw in a lot of onion, garlic, bell pepper and jalapeno. Proceed to sauté them until they get slightly tender.
2. Put the chicken into the pan. Cook till you can no longer see pink color on the outside part of the chicken.
3. After that, add white beans, diced tomatoes and chicken broth and stir.
4. Finally, mix well with chili powder, cumin, oregano, salt, and pepper.
5. For about 45 minutes to an hour, simmer covered for 45 minutes or until desired consistency is achieved, stirring occasionally; bring chili to a boil, then reduce heat to low.
6. Taste your chili as per how tasty you want it. Serve warm with cilantro cheese sour cream or avocado toppings.

**Nutrition (per serving):**

Calories: 350 kcal Protein: 35 g Carbohydrates: 35 g Fiber: 10 g Healthy Fats: 7 g

# 9. Chicken Kabobs

**Prep Time: 20 minutes Cook Time: 10-15 minutes Servings: 4**

## Ingredients

- 1 ½ pounds boneless, skinless chicken breasts cut into 1-inch cubes
- 2 bell peppers, cut into 1-inch pieces
- 1 large red onion, cut into 1-inch pieces
- 1 zucchini, sliced into 1/2-inch rounds
- 1/2 cup of olive oil
- 3 tbsp lemon juice
- 2 garlic cloves, minced
- 1 tsp dried oregano
- 1 tsp paprika
- Salt and pepper, to taste
- Wooden or metal skewers

## Instructions

1. Whisk together olive oil, minced garlic, lemon juice, paprika, oregano, salt, and pepper in a bowl.
2. Marinate the chicken cubes in it, ensuring they are well covered. You may refrigerate for 1 or more hours with the cover on for more decadent tastes.
3. Preheat an outdoor grill to a medium-high heat position. If using wooden skewers, make sure to soak them in water for at least 30 minutes to prevent burning.
4. Alternating between meat and vegetables, thread marinated chicken, zucchini, bell peppers, and red onion onto skewers.
5. Grill for 10 – 15 minutes, turning occasionally until the chicken is done and the vegetables turn tender, after placing the kabobs on a preheated grill.
6. Take off from oven and serve Kabobs hot.

**Nutrition (per serving):**

Calories: 400 kcal Protein: 35 g Carbohydrates: 15 g Fiber: 3 g Healthy Fats: 20 g

# 10. Chicken Stir-Fry

**Prep Time: 15 minutes Cook Time: 15 minutes Servings: 4**

## Ingredients

- 1 ½ pounds boneless, skinless chicken breasts, thinly sliced
- 3 cups of mixed vegetables
- 1 onion, sliced
- 2 garlic cloves, minced
- 2 tbsp vegetable oil
- 1/4 cup of low-sodium soy sauce
- 2 tbsp oyster sauce (optional)
- 1 tbsp cornstarch
- 1/2 cup of chicken broth or water
- 1 tsp ginger, grated
- Salt and pepper, to taste

Optional: sesame seeds, green onions for garnish

## Instructions

1. Combine soy sauce, oyster sauce, cornstarch and chicken broth in a small bowl. Leave it aside.
2. Heat 1 tablespoon of oil in a large skillet or wok over medium-high heat. Add salt and pepper to the chicken slices. Add these to the skillet and cook till done through, browned slightly by stirring constantly. After removing the chicken from the pan, set aside.
3. Add the remaining oil to the skillet. Stir fry onions and garlic for one minute. When the vegetables are tender but still crisp, include mixed vegetables & ginger during stir-frying.
4. Mix with all ingredients in the above step before serving
5. Put the back chicken into the vegetable mixture
6. Pour sauce over the chicken-vegetable mixture at this stage, then keep stirring until it thickens.
7. You can garnish this hot stir-fry with sesame seeds as you like or/and cut green onions.

**Nutrition (per serving)**

Calories: 300 kcal Protein: 35 g Carbohydrates: 15 g Fiber: 3 g Healthy Fats: 10 g

# 11. Salad with Grilled Chicken

**Prep Time: 15 minutes Cook Time: 10 minutes Servings: 4**

## Ingredients

- 4 boneless, skinless chicken breasts
- 8 cups of mixed salad greens
- 1 cup of cherry tomatoes, halved
- 1 cucumber, sliced
- 1 red bell pepper, sliced
- 1/4 red onion, thinly sliced
- 1 avocado, sliced (optional)
- 1/4 cup of balsamic vinaigrette
- 2 tbsp olive oil
- Salt and pepper, to taste

Optional garnishes: crumbled feta or goat cheese, nuts, or croutons

## Instructions

1. Put some black pepper and salt on the chicken breasts. Place your grill over medium-high heat until it gets hot. 1 tablespoon of olive oil can be used for brushing.
2. Grill the chicken for about five minutes or until done (internal temperature of 165°F/75°C). Take it off the grill, then rest it for a few minutes. Slice into strips after that.
3. If desired, combine salad greens, cherry tomatoes, cucumber, bell pepper, red onion, and avocado in a large bowl.
4. Place grilled sliced chicken atop the salad.
5. Pour balsamic vinaigrette over the salad.
6. Gently toss salad to mix. Serve immediately with optional toppings, including cheese, nuts or croutons as garnish.

**Nutrition (per serving):**

Calories: 350 kcal Protein: 30 g Carbohydrates: 15 g Fiber: 6 g Healthy Fats: 20 g

# 12. Roasted Balsamic Chicken



## Ingredients

- 4 boneless, skinless chicken breasts
- 1/4 cup of balsamic vinegar
- 2 tbsp olive oil
- 2 garlic cloves, minced
- 1 tsp dried thyme
- 1 tsp dried rosemary
- Salt and pepper, to taste

Optional: vegetables like bell peppers, onions, and zucchini for roasting

## Instructions

1. Combine balsamic vinegar, olive oil, minced garlic, thyme, rosemary, salt, and pepper in a large bowl. Dip chicken breasts into the marinade until coated well. Cover and place in the refrigerator for at least half an hour, but if possible, a couple of hours.
2. Turn on your oven to 375°F (190°C).
3. Put the marinated chicken breasts into a baking pan. If serving with vegetables, mix them with some olive oil, salt, and pepper and arrange them around the chicken.
4. Roast at these temperatures for 30-35 minutes or until the temperature inside the chicken reaches 165°F (75°C).
5. Allow the chicken to rest for a few moments before eating it.

**Nutrition (per serving):**

Calories: 300 kcal Protein: 35 g Carbohydrates: 5 g Fiber: 1 g Healthy Fats: 10 g

# 13. Spicy Turkey Stir Fry

**Prep Time: 15 minutes Cook Time: 10 minutes Servings: 4**

## Ingredients

- 1 pound ground turkey
- 2 cups of broccoli florets
- 1 red bell pepper, sliced
- 1 carrot, julienned
- 1 onion, sliced
- 2 garlic cloves, minced
- 1 tbsp fresh ginger, minced
- 2 tbsp vegetable oil
- 2 tbsp soy sauce (low-sodium)
- 2 tbsp oyster sauce (optional)
- 1 tbsp chilli garlic sauce or sriracha
- 1 tsp cornstarch
- Salt and pepper, to taste
- Optional garnishes: green onions, sesame seeds

## Instructions

1. Put 1 tablespoon of oil in a big frying pan or wok and then heat. Add the beef to it, sprinkle with salt and pepper and cook until browned and done. Take out the chicken from this pan and set aside.
2. Drop off some remaining oil in your saucepan. Add broccoli, bell pepper, carrot, onion, garlic, and ginger. These vegetables should be stir-fried until they are tender yet keep their crispiness.
3. In another bowl, combine soy sauce, oyster sauce, and chili garlic sauce together with the cornstarch mixture.
4. Put the cooked turkey back into the pan that contains vegetables. After pouring the sauce over it, stir-fry for about 2-3 minutes until it becomes thick and coats the ingredients in that dish.
5. Serve hot and garnished using green onions and sesame seeds if you wish.

**Nutrition (per serving):**

Calories: 250 kcal Protein: 25 g Carbohydrates: 15 g Fiber: 3 g Healthy Fats: 10 g

# 14. Pulled Chicken BBQ Sandwich

**Prep Time: 20 minutes Cook Time: 1 hour Servings: 4**

## Ingredients

- 4 boneless, skinless chicken breasts
- 1 cup of barbecue sauce
- 1 tbsp olive oil
- 1 small onion, finely chopped
- 2 garlic cloves, minced
- 1/2 cup of chicken broth
- 4 sandwich buns, split and toasted
- Optional toppings: coleslaw, pickles, extra barbecue sauce
- Salt and pepper, to taste

## Instructions

1. Put salt and pepper on the chicken breasts. Heat olive oil in a large pot over medium heat. Put the chicken in and let it turn brown on both sides. After that, add garlic and chopped onion around the chicken and fry until they become soft. Pour the chicken broth into the pot, cover it and let it simmer for nearly 1 hour. The chicken is done once it is so tender as to fall apart when pulled by a fork.
2. Take the chicken out of the pot and use two forks to shred it.
3. Put shredded chicken back into the pan. Stir barbecue sauce into the mixture. Also, cook at a low temperature for 10 minutes to blend all flavors with the meat.
4. Spread some pulled chicken over each toasted half of the sandwich bun. Place coleslaw, if preferred, on top of the pickle or extra BBQ sauce on top if desired.
5. Finally, put together sandwiches by placing pieces of buns on top of them before serving immediately.

**Nutrition (per serving):**

Calories: 400 kcal Protein: 35 g Carbohydrates: 45 g Fiber: 3 g Healthy Fats: 12 g

# 15. Grilled Chicken Breast Sandwich

**Prep Time: 15 minutes Cook Time: 10 minutes Servings: 4**

## Ingredients

- 4 boneless, skinless chicken breasts
- 4 sandwich buns
- 1 tbsp olive oil
- 1 tsp garlic powder
- 1 tsp paprika
- Salt and pepper, to taste
- 4 lettuce leaves
- 1 tomato, sliced
- 1 red onion, thinly sliced

## Instructions

1. Preheat your grill or grill pan to medium-high heat.
2. Olive oil should be used to brush the chicken breasts. They are then seasoned with garlic powder, salt, paprika and pepper.
3. It is about five minutes on each side of grilling the chicken breast until it's fully cooked. After taking them out of the grill, let them sit for some time.
4. If desired, you can slightly toast the sandwich buns on the grill.
5. Place one leaf lettuce in each bun at the bottom; add grilled chicken breast followed by tomato slices, red onions, and mayonnaise, mustard, and ketchup toppings if desired.
6. Finish the sandwiches by closing them with the top halves of the buns. If preferred, serve with pickles or coleslaw on a side.

**Nutrition (per serving):**

Calories: 350 kcal Protein: 30 g Carbohydrates: 35 g Fiber: 4 g Healthy Fats: 12 g

# 16. Teriyaki Chicken with Jasmine Rice

**Prep Time: 15 minutes Cook Time: 25 minutes Servings: 4**

## Ingredients

- 4 boneless, skinless chicken breasts
- 1 cup of jasmine rice
- 2 cups of water
- 1/2 cup of teriyaki sauce
- 2 tbsp honey
- 2 garlic cloves, minced
- 1 tbsp fresh ginger, grated
- 2 tbsp vegetable oil
- Salt and pepper, to taste

## Instructions

1. You will need to wash the jasmine rice in cold water until it is clear. Boil the rice with two cups of water on a pan. Turn down the flame, cover it, and boil it for 18-20 minutes or until it is cooked and water has been absorbed.
2. Blend teriyaki sauce, honey, garlic minced, and ginger grated in a tiny bowl.
3. Salt and pepper the chicken breasts. Put the vegetable oil in a large skillet set over medium-high heat. Cook the chicken on each side for about five to seven minutes until golden brown and correctly done.
4. In your frying pan, pour your mixture of teriyaki sauce all over your chicken, then simmer for a few minutes while flipping it constantly so the sauce coats it well.
5. Carve up the chicken and place it on top of cooked jasmine rice. If desired, sprinkle with sesame seeds and green onions. This meal can be balanced when accompanied by steamed broccoli or stir-fried vegetables.

**Nutrition (per serving):**

Calories: 450 kcal Protein: 35 g Carbohydrates: 55 g Fiber: 2 g Healthy Fats: 10 g

# 17. Grilled Chicken Breast with Roasted Vegetables

**Prep Time: 20 minutes Cook Time: 30 minutes Servings: 4**

## Ingredients

- 4 boneless, skinless chicken breasts
- 2 bell peppers (any color), cut into chunks
- 1 zucchini, sliced
- 1 red onion, cut into wedges
- 1 cup of cherry tomatoes
- 1/4 cup of olive oil, divided
- 2 tbsp balsamic vinegar
- 2 garlic cloves, minced
- 1 tsp dried thyme
- 1 tsp dried rosemary
- Salt and pepper, to taste
- Optional: fresh herbs (like parsley or basil) for garnish

## Instructions

1. Place 1 minced garlic clove, thyme, rosemary, salt and pepper in a mixing bowl and add balsamic vinegar and olive oil. Ensure that the chicken breasts are coated well by applying the mixture. Keep for at least 15 minutes, but preferably more.
2. Preheat the grill to medium-high heat and then preheat its oven to 400°F (200°C).
3. Combine bell peppers, zucchini, red onion and cherry tomatoes with remaining olive oil mixed with garlic, thyme and rosemary. Season with salt and pepper.
4. Take a baking sheet and spread vegetables on it in one layer. Put them on the lower rack of an already heated oven for around 20-25 minutes until they get tenderized and slightly charred.
5. Grill marinated chicken breasts for about six to seven minutes per side until they are cooked through (165°F or 75°C). Allow to rest for a few minutes before slicing.
6. Serve sliced grilled chicken accompanied with roasted vegetables on the side. If desired, garnish with fresh herbs.

**Nutrition (per serving):**

Calories: 400 kcal Protein: 35 g Carbohydrates: 20 g Fiber: 5 g Healthy Fats: 15 g

# 18. Olive Chicken

**Prep Time: 15 minutes Cook Time: 30 minutes Servings: 4**

## Ingredients

- 4 boneless, skinless chicken breasts
- 1 cup of mixed olives, pitted and sliced
- 1 large onion, chopped
- 2 garlic cloves, minced
- 1 can (14.5 oz) diced tomatoes
- 1/2 cup of chicken broth
- 2 tbsp olive oil
- 1 tsp dried thyme
- 1 tsp dried rosemary
- Salt and pepper, to taste
- Optional: lemon zest, fresh parsley for garnish

## Instructions

1. Place the chicken breasts on a plate and season with salt and pepper. Heat the olive oil in a large skillet over medium-high heat. Add chicken; cook for 4 minutes on each side or until browned. Remove chicken from pan and set aside.
2. Using the same skillet, add chopped onions and minced garlic. Cook until the onions are soft and transparent.
3. Combine olives, diced tomatoes (with juice), chicken broth, thyme and rosemary in that order. Bring mixture to a simmer.
4. Arrange the cooked chicken breast in a serving tray, then drizzle with sauce and top with olive pieces. Cover it, then simmer it for about 20 minutes or until the meat is tender enough. Serve hot, garnished with lemon zest and parsley if you like adding such ingredients.

**Nutrition (per serving)**

Calories: 350 kcal Protein: 35 g Carbohydrates: 15 g Fiber: 3 g Healthy Fats: 20 g

## 1. Avocado and Salmon Salad

**Prep Time: 15 minutes Cook Time: 0 minutes Servings: 2**

### Ingredients

- 2 medium-sized ripe avocados, peeled, pitted, and sliced
- 200 grams of smoked salmon, thinly sliced
- 2 cups of mixed greens
- 1 small red onion, thinly sliced
- 1/4 cup of capers
- 2 tbsp olive oil
- 1 tbsp lemon juice
- Salt and pepper to taste
- Fresh dill or parsley for garnish (optional)

### Instructions

1. Combine the mixed greens, sliced red onion, and capers in a large bowl.
2. Place smoked salmon slices on top of the greens, then place avocado slices on top.
3. Whisk together olive oil, lemon juice, salt and pepper in a small bowl. Taste and adjust seasoning.
4. Drizzle over salad dressing, and toss everything without breaking the avocado pieces.
5. To garnish, use dill or parsley if you can find it. It should be served immediately to keep its freshness.

**Nutrition (per serving)**

Calories: 450 kcal Protein: 25 g Carbohydrates: 20 g Fats: 35 g Fiber: 10 g

# 2. Rustic Scallops with Coriander and Lime

**Prep Time: 10 minutes Cook Time: 6-8 minutes Servings: 2**

## Ingredients

- 400 grams of fresh scallops, cleaned and patted dry
- 2 tbsp olive oil
- 2 cloves of garlic, minced
- 1 tsp ground coriander
- Zest and juice of 1 lime
- Salt and pepper to taste
- Fresh coriander (cilantro) leaves for garnish
- Lime wedges for serving

## Instructions

1. Season the scallops with ground coriander, salt, and pepper in a bowl.
2. Heat the olive oil in a big skillet over medium-high heat.
3. Place a single layer of scallops in the skillet. Fry 2 to 3 minutes on each side until they are cooked through and have a golden crust. Add the minced garlic to the pan halfway through.
4. After the scallops are done, take the skillet off the burner and carefully mix the scallops in the lime juice and zest.
5. Serve the scallops with lime wedges and fresh coriander leaves on the side.

**Nutrition (per serving):**

Calories: 300 kcal Protein: 28 g Carbohydrates: 5 g Fats: 14 g Fiber: 1 g

# 3. Shrimp Shiitake Pot Stickers



## Ingredients

- 300 grams of shrimp, peeled, deveined, and finely chopped
- 1 cup of shiitake mushrooms, finely chopped
- 2 green onions, finely chopped
- 1 tbsp soy sauce (low sodium)
- 1 tsp sesame oil
- 1/2 tsp ginger, grated
- 1 garlic clove, minced
- Salt and pepper to taste
- 24 wonton wrappers
- 2 tbsp vegetable oil for frying
- Water for steaming
- Dipping sauce

## Instructions

1. Add the chopped shrimp, green onions, ginger, garlic, salt and pepper in a bowl. Mix well.
2. Put some fillings on the middle of each wonton wrapper; moisten the edges with water, fold them in half, and press to seal, ensuring no air pockets.
3. Heat 1 tablespoon of vegetable oil in a large skillet over medium heat. Put half the pot stickers into the skillet and cook until their bottoms become golden brown (around 2 minutes). After that, add ¼ cup of water into the skillet, cover it, then steam for about 5 minutes or until all water has evaporated & dumplings are cooked through. Repeat with remaining pot stickers.
4. Serve hot with dipping sauce on the side.

**Nutrition (per serving)**

Calories: 300 kcal Protein: 20 g Carbohydrates: 25 g Fats: 12 g Fiber: 2 g

# 4. Protein-Packed Paella

**Prep Time: 20 minutes Cook Time: 40 minutes Servings: 4**

## Ingredients

- 200 grams boneless, skinless chicken breast, cut into bite-sized pieces
- 200 grams of shrimp, peeled and deveined
- 200 grams mussels, cleaned and de-bearded
- 1 cup of short-grain paella rice
- 1 onion, finely chopped
- 2 cloves garlic, minced
- 1 red bell pepper, sliced
- 1 cup of canned diced tomatoes
- 3 cups of low-sodium chicken broth
- 1 tsp smoked paprika
- 1/2 tsp saffron threads
- 2 tbsp olive oil
- Salt and pepper to taste
- Fresh parsley and lemon wedges for garnish

## Instructions

1. A large skillet or paella pan should be heated with one tablespoon of olive oil on medium heat. Brown the chicken in it, season it with salt and pepper, then remove and set it aside. Similarly, do so with the shrimp.
2. The remaining olive oil should be poured into the pan. Soften onion, garlic, and bell pepper by sautéing them.
3. Stir the rice with smoked paprika and saffron so that the rice is coated with these spices. A few minutes later, add chopped tomatoes.
4. Pour in chicken broth and simmer before reducing heat to low. Leave uncovered for about 20 minutes until rice is nearly done.
5. Put chicken, shrimp, and mussels into rice; cover the pan. Cook for another ten to fifteen minutes until the mussels have opened up, and the rice is tender.
6. Remove any unopened mussels. Sprinkle some fresh parsley leaves on top, then serve alongside lemon wedges.

**Nutrition (per serving):**

Calories: 400 kcal Protein: 35 g Carbohydrates: 40 g Fats: 12 g Fiber: 3 g

# 5. Grilled Tuna Teriyaki

**Prep Time: 15 minutes Cook Time: 6-8 minutes Servings: 4**

## Ingredients

- 4 tuna steaks (about 150 grams each)
- 1/4 cup of low-sodium soy sauce
- 2 tbsp rice vinegar
- 1 tbsp honey
- 1 garlic clove, minced
- 1 tsp fresh ginger, grated
- 1 tsp sesame oil
- Sesame seeds for garnish
- Green onions, thinly sliced for garnish

## Instructions

1. Whisk together soy sauce, rice vinegar, honey, garlic, ginger and sesame oil in a bowl. Take the tuna steaks to a shallow bowl and pour over them the marinade. Allow them to marinate in the fridge for at least 30 minutes, turning once.
2. Preheat your grill to medium-high heat.
3. Grill tuna for about 3-4 minutes on each side for medium-rare or longer if you like it cooked better done.
4. While the tuna is grilling, pour the remaining marinade into a small saucepan. Bring to a boil, then simmer over low heat until slightly thickened.
5. Place grilled tuna on plates; drizzle with teriyaki sauce; sprinkle with sesame seeds and green onions.

**Nutrition (per serving)**

Calories: 300 kcal Protein: 30 g Carbohydrates: 10 g Fats: 7 g Fiber: Less than 1 g

# 6. Tuna Salad Sandwich on Whole-Wheat Bread

**Prep Time: 10 minutes Cook Time: 0 minutes Servings: 4 sandwiches**

## Ingredients

- 2 cans (about 120 grams each) of tuna in water, drained
- 1/4 cup of low-fat mayonnaise
- 1 celery stalk, finely chopped
- 2 tbsp red onion, finely chopped
- 1 tbsp fresh lemon juice
- 1 tsp Dijon mustard
- Salt and pepper to taste
- 8 slices of whole-wheat bread
- Lettuce leaves
- Tomato slices

## Instructions

1. In a bowl, combine the drained tuna with low-fat mayonnaise, celery that has been chopped up, red onions, lemon juice, Dijon mustard salt and pepper. Stir until well combined.
2. Lay out 4 slices of whole-wheat bread. Spread the tuna mixture evenly among these slices. Add lettuce leaves and tomato slices on top of the tuna mixture.
3. Place the remaining slices of bread on top. Press together lightly to hold in place.
4. Cut sandwiches in half and serve at once, or wrap them up.

**Nutrition (per sandwich):**

Calories: 300 kcal Protein: 25 g Carbohydrates: 30 g Fats: 5 g Fiber: 6 g

# 7. Salmon with Quinoa and Roasted Veggies

**Prep Time: 15 minutes Cook Time: 25-30 minutes Servings: 4**

## Ingredients

- 4 salmon fillets (about 150 grams each)
- 1 cup of quinoa
- 2 cups of water or low-sodium vegetable broth
- 1 zucchini, sliced into half-moons
- 1 red bell pepper, cut into strips
- 1 yellow bell pepper, cut into strips
- 1 small red onion, sliced
- 2 tbsp olive oil
- 1 lemon, zest, and juice
- Salt and pepper to taste
- Fresh herbs (like parsley or dill) for garnish

## Instructions

1. Preheat your oven to 200°C (400°F).
2. Mix the zucchini, bell peppers, and red onions with one tablespoon of olive oil, salt, and pepper. Transfer them to a baking sheet and then bake in an oven for 20 minutes until they become tender and slightly caramelized.
3. Cold rinse quinoa under running water. Boil water or vegetable broth in a saucepan. Add the quinoa, lower heat, cover and cook for around 15 minutes or until all the liquid disappears. Fluff with a fork.
4. At the same time as roasting vegetables and boiling quinoa, sprinkle some salt, pepper and lemon rind on the salmon fillets. On medium-high heat in a skillet, add the remaining olive oil. Cook salmon on each side for approximately 4-5 minutes, or when done to your liking, finish by squeezing fresh lemon juice.
5. Serve up plates containing roasted vegetables garnished with quinoa. Over each place, salmon fillet. Decorate using fresh herbs, and have a piece of lemon to eat alongside it.

**Nutrition (per serving):**

Calories: 450 kcal Protein: 35 g Carbohydrates: 35 g Fats: 20 g Fiber: 7 g

# 8. Parmesan-Crusted Salmon

**Prep Time: 10 minutes Cook Time: 15 minutes Servings: 4**

## Ingredients

- 4 salmon fillets
- 1/2 cup of grated Parmesan cheese
- 1/4 cup of whole wheat breadcrumbs
- 1 garlic clove, minced
- 1 tbsp fresh parsley, chopped
- Zest of 1 lemon
- 2 tbsp olive oil
- Salt and pepper to taste
- Lemon wedges for serving

## Instructions

1. Preheat your oven to 200°C (400°F).
2. In a bowl, combine the cheese, which is grated Parmesan, bread crumbs, whole wheat, minced garlic, fresh leaf parsley, chopped lemon zest, and lemon zest.
3. Line the baking sheet with parchment paper. Place salmon fillets on it. Rub olive oil over each, then season with pepper and salt.
4. Form crusts by patting Parmesan onto the top side of each salmon fillet.
5. Put in a preheated oven for around 12-15 minutes until the salmon becomes opaque and the topping is browned to crispy.
6. Place lemon wedges next to the salmon covered in Parmesan.

**Nutrition (per serving)**

Calories: 350 kcal Protein: 30 g Carbohydrates: 10 g Fats: 20 g Fiber: 2 g

# 9. Garlic and Herb Seared Salmon

**Prep Time: 10 minutes Cook Time: 10 minutes Servings: 4**

## Ingredients

- 4 salmon fillets
- 2 tbsp olive oil
- 2 garlic cloves, minced
- 1 tbsp fresh rosemary, finely chopped
- 1 tbsp fresh thyme, finely chopped
- 1 tbsp fresh parsley, finely chopped
- Zest of 1 lemon
- Salt and pepper to taste
- Lemon wedges for serving

## Instructions

1. Mix minced garlic, rosemary, thyme, parsley, and lemon zest in a small bowl.
2. Salt and pepper the salmon fillets. Spread herb mixture onto each fillet to coat them well.
3. Heat olive oil in a big frying pan over medium-high heat.
4. Put salmon fillets into skillet with skin side down. Cook until the skin is crispy for about 5 minutes. Now flip the fish carefully and cook for 4-5 minutes until it becomes as done as you want.
5. Serve salmon at once and garnish with lemon wedges.

**Nutrition (per serving)**

Calories: 300 kcal Protein: 28 g Carbohydrates: 2 g Fats: 18 g Fiber: 1 g

# 10. Shrimp Creole

**Prep Time: 15 minutes Cook Time: 25 minutes Servings: 4**

## Ingredients

- 500 grams of shrimp, peeled and deveined
- 1 tbsp olive oil
- 1 large onion, chopped
- 1 green bell pepper, chopped
- 1 red bell pepper, chopped
- 3 cloves of garlic, minced
- 1 can (400 grams) of diced tomatoes
- 1/2 cup of low-sodium chicken or vegetable broth
- 2 tbsp tomato paste
- 1 tsp paprika
- 1/2 tsp cayenne pepper
- 1 tsp dried oregano
- 1 tsp dried thyme
- Salt and pepper to taste
- 2 tbsp fresh parsley, chopped
- Cooked brown rice or cauliflower rice for serving

## Instructions

1. Heat the olive oil in a big frying pan over moderate heat. Then, you can chop onions, bell peppers, and garlic and fry them until they are soft, which is about 5 minutes.
2. Put in the diced tomatoes whilst stirring, and add their broth (can be chicken or vegetable), tomato paste, cayenne pepper, paprika, oregano, and thyme. Adjust your salt and pepper seasoning, and then start to simmer it.
3. Simmer for about 15 minutes so that all the flavors may intermingle together.
4. Stir it continuously while you add shrimp to your skillet. Wait about 5-6 minutes or until it looks pinkish and cooked through (shrimp).
5. Then, mix the fresh parsley with other ingredients where necessary.
6. For a low-carb alternative, serve Shrimp Creole over cooked brown rice or cauliflower rice.

**Nutrition (per serving)**

Calories: 250 kcal Protein: 30 g Carbohydrates: 15 g Fats: 8 g Fiber: 3 g

# 11. Super Human Sea Bass with Sizzling Spices

**Prep Time: 10 minutes Cook Time: 12 minutes Servings: 4**

## Ingredients

- 4 sea bass fillets
- 1 tbsp olive oil
- 1 tsp paprika
- 1/2 tsp ground cumin
- 1/2 tsp garlic powder
- 1/4 tsp cayenne pepper (adjust to taste)
- 1/2 tsp dried oregano
- Salt and black pepper to taste
- Lemon wedges for serving
- Fresh parsley or cilantro for garnish

## Instructions

1. Mix the paprika, cumin powder, garlic salt, crushed chilies, dried marjoram, sea salt and black pepper in a small bowl.
2. Spread the spice mixture on both sides of the fillets uniformly.
3. Heat olive oil over medium-hot flame in a large skillet. Add fillets and cook for 5-6 minutes per side until the fork easily flakes fish.
4. Serve with lemon wedges and garnish with fresh parsley or coriander.

**Nutrition (per serving):**

Calories: 250 kcal Protein: 28 g Carbohydrates: 2 g Fats: 12 g Fiber: 1 g

# 12. Bourbon Lime Salmon

**Prep Time: 10 minutes Cook Time: 10-12 minutes Servings: 4**

## Ingredients

- 4 salmon fillets
- 1/4 cup of bourbon
- 2 tbsp soy sauce (low sodium)
- 1 tbsp honey
- Juice and zest of 1 lime
- 1 garlic clove, minced
- 1 tsp fresh ginger, grated
- 2 tbsp olive oil
- Salt and pepper to taste
- Fresh lime slices for garnish

## Instructions

1. Mix bourbon, honey, soy sauce, lime juice, zest, grated ginger, and minced garlic in a bowl. Place the salmon fillets in a shallow bowl or a zip-lock bag and pour the marinade over them. Let them marinate in the refrigerator for at least 30 minutes.
2. Preheat your grill to medium-high heat, or heat a skillet with olive oil on medium-high.
3. Salt and Pepper the salmon after removing it from the marinade just before grilling or placing it on the pan and cook it for about 5-6 minutes on each side until the desired done-ness is reached.
4. While the salmon is cooking, transfer any remaining marinade into a small bowl. Pour it into an empty pan and boil; then simmer over low heat until slightly thickened because this can make a glaze for salmon.
5. Serve cooked fish on plates; drizzle some reduced marinade over (if used) and garnish with slices of fresh lime.

**Nutrition (per serving):**

Calories: 350 kcal Protein: 28 g Carbohydrates: 10 g Fats: 20 g Fiber: 1 g

# 13. Brawny Baked Haddock with Spinach

**Prep Time: 10 minutes Cook Time: 20 minutes Servings: 4**

## Ingredients

- 4 haddock fillets
- 2 tbsp olive oil
- 2 cloves garlic, minced
- 4 cups of fresh spinach leaves
- 1 lemon, zest and juice
- 1 tsp dried thyme
- Salt and pepper to taste
- Lemon slices for garnish

## Instructions

1. Preheat your oven to 190°C (375°F).
2. Over medium heat in a large skillet, wait for the pan to warm up with one tbsp of olive oil. Cook garlic, stirring it frequently until they become fragrant; around sixty seconds. As shown below, salt and pepper can be used to season spinach to become soft when cooked for three or four minutes.
3. Mix lemon zest, thyme, salt and pepper in a small bowl before using this mixture to rub over haddock fillets.
4. Next, place wilted spinach in a baking pan, followed by seasoned haddock fillets on top of the spinach bed. Finish with remaining olive oil and lemon juice.
5. Preheat oven and bake the haddock for 12 – 15 minutes; more accurately, check if the fish is ready by piercing it with a fork till it flakes easily.
6. To garnish, serve baked haddock and spinach with thin slices of lemon.

**Nutrition (per serving):**

Calories: 250 kcal Protein: 30 g Carbohydrates: 5 g Fats: 12 g Fiber: 3 g

# 14. Tangy Trout

**Prep Time: 10 minutes Cook Time: 10 minutes Servings: 4**

## Ingredients

- 4 trout fillets
- 1 lemon, zest and juice
- 2 tbsp Dijon mustard
- 1 tbsp honey
- 2 cloves garlic, minced
- 2 tbsp olive oil
- Salt and pepper to taste
- Fresh herbs for garnish

## Instructions

1. Mix lemon zest and juice, honey, Dijon mustard, minced garlic, and 1 tbsp olive oil in a small bowl; season with salt and pepper.
2. Place the trout fillets inside a shallow bowl or resalable plastic bag. Pour the marinade over the trout fillets to coat them properly. Then refrigerate until it has marinated for at least thirty minutes.
3. Preheat your grill to medium-high heat, or heat a non-stick skillet with the remaining olive oil over medium-high heat.
4. Take out fish from the marinade and let any extra liquid run. If they have skin, put the fillets onto the grill/skillet skin-side down. Cook for about five minutes on each side until the fish is cooked and flakes easily.
5. Serve immediately with fresh herbs as a garnish for your trout.

**Nutrition (per serving)**

Calories: 300 kcal Protein: 28 g Carbohydrates: 10 g Fats: 15 g Fiber: 1 g

# 15. Cod with Bacon, Red Onion, and Kale

**Prep Time: 10 minutes Cook Time: 20 minutes Servings: 4**

## Ingredients

- 4 cod fillets
- 4 slices of bacon, chopped
- 1 large red onion, thinly sliced
- 2 cups of kale, stems removed and leaves chopped
- 2 cloves of garlic, minced
- 1 tbsp olive oil
- Salt and pepper to taste
- Lemon wedges for serving

## Instructions

1. In a large frying pan, cook the diced bacon until crispy over medium heat. Remove the bacon from the skillet, keeping the fat in it.
2. Put the red onion in the pan and cook for five minutes until soft. Add kale and garlic and let it cook for 5 more minutes or until kale is wilted. Season to taste with salt and pepper. Take out of the pan.
3. Next, add one tbsp of olive oil to this same pan and then put cod fillets into it after sprinkling them with salt & pepper; fry for about 4-5 minutes on each side or until fish flakes properly when tested using a fork.
4. Put back into skillet with cod, heating through with bacon and onion mixture made above with kale.
5. Serve hot cod topped with bacon, onions and kale. Accompany with lemon wedges.

**Nutrition (per serving):**

Calories: 300 kcal Protein: 30 g Carbohydrates: 10 g Fats: 15 g Fiber: 3 g

# 16. Lemon Dill Salmon

**Prep Time: 10 minutes Cook Time: 20 minutes Servings: 4**

## Ingredients

- 4 salmon fillets
- 2 lemons, one sliced and one juiced
- 2 tbsp fresh dill, chopped
- 2 tbsp olive oil
- 2 garlic cloves, minced
- Salt and pepper to taste
- Additional dill sprigs for garnish

## Instructions

1. Preheat your oven to 200°C (400°F).
2. Arrange the salmon fillets in a baking pan, then sprinkle with salt, pepper, minced garlic and chopped dill.
3. Drizzle olive oil and lemon juice all over the salmon. Then, place slices of lemon on top and around these fish.
4. You should bake the fish for 15-20 minutes in a preheated oven until it flakes when poked with a fork.
5. Garnish the salmons with a few more sprigs of fresh dill before serving.

**Nutrition (per serving):**

Calories: 300 kcal Protein: 28 g Carbohydrates: 4 g Fats: 18 g Fiber: Less than 1 g Sodium: Low

# 17. Healthy Fish and Chips

**Prep Time: 20 minutes Cook Time: 40 minutes Servings: 4**

## Ingredients

For the Fish:

- 4 white fish fillets
- 1/2 cup of whole wheat flour
- 2 eggs, beaten
- 1 cup of whole-grain breadcrumbs
- 1 tsp paprika
- Salt and pepper to taste

For the Chips:

- 4 large potatoes, peeled and cut into wedges
- 2 tbsp olive oil
- Salt and pepper to taste
- Optional herbs

## Instructions

1. Preheat your oven to 220°C (425°F) and prepare two baking sheets with parchment paper.
2. Toss in olive oil, salt, pepper and any other desired herbs. Put them all on one of the baking sheets without piling them up. Bake for 35-40 minutes, turning halfway through until they are golden and crispy.
3. Prepare three plates: one with flour, another with beaten eggs, and a third with breadcrumbs mixed with colored salt and ground red peppers. First, roll each fish fillet into flour, then the egg mixture, and then gauge it in bread crumbs.
4. Put the breaded fish onto the second sheet. Bake this for 12-15 minutes to cook fish until cooked through and golden crust is obtained.
5. Combine the fried fish with chips made in an oven on a plate. For instance, peas or salad can be served as side dishes for a balanced meal.

**Nutrition (Per Serving):**

Calories: 450 kcal Protein: 25 g Carbohydrates: 60 g Fats: 15 g Fiber: 8 g

# 18. Sea Bass with Vegetables

**Prep Time: 15 minutes Cook Time: 25 minutes Servings: 4**

## Ingredients

- 4 sea bass fillets
- 1 zucchini, sliced
- 1 red bell pepper, cut into strips
- 1 yellow bell pepper, cut into strips
- 1 small red onion, sliced
- 2 tbsp olive oil
- 1 lemon, sliced
- 2 cloves of garlic, minced
- Salt and pepper to taste
- Fresh herbs (like thyme or parsley) for garnish

## Instructions

1. Set your oven to 200°C (400°F).
2. Throw one tbsp of olive oil, salt and pepper into the sliced zucchini, bell peppers and red onion to mix them. Then, spread over a baking sheet.
3. Also, rub minced garlic, salt and pepper with the remaining olive oil on the sea bass fillets. Top with lemon slices.
4. Atop the vegetable layer on a baking sheet sit the sea bass fillets. In a preheated oven, bake for approximately 20-25 minutes until the fish is cooked through and the vegetables are tender.
5. Garnish it with fresh herbs before serving it hot.

**Nutrition (Per Serving)**

Calories: 270 kcal Protein: 28 g Carbohydrates: 15 g Fats: 12 g Fiber: 3 g

## 1. Salmon Chickpea Salad

**Prep Time: 15 minutes Cook Time: 0 minutes Servings: 4**

## Ingredients

- 2 cans of drained salmon
- 1 can of chickpeas, rinsed and drained
- 1 large cucumber, diced
- 1 red bell pepper, diced
- 1/2 red onion, finely chopped
- 1/4 cup of fresh parsley, chopped
- 2 tbsp olive oil
- Juice of 1 lemon
- 1 tsp Dijon mustard
- Salt and pepper to taste

Optional: crumbled feta cheese or avocado slices for topping

## Instructions

1. Seasoned with parsley, red onion, bell pepper, cucumber and chickpeas, the salmon is drained and poured into a large bowl.
2. The other dressing ingredients include salt, Dijon mustard, lemon juice and olive oil mixed in a small bowl.
3. Mixing the salad mixture with some dressing before putting it on a dish so that it becomes even.
4. Apart from crumbled feta cheese or avocado slices, which may be added for enhanced taste and richness, you will be served this salad in bowls.

**Nutrition (Per Serving):**

Calories: 350 kcal Protein: 20 g Carbohydrates: 25 g Fats: 10 g Fiber: 6 g

# 2. Cabbage Slaw

**Prep Time: 15 minutes Cook Time: 0 minutes Servings: 4**

## Ingredients

- 1/2 head of green cabbage, thinly sliced
- 1/2 head of red cabbage, thinly sliced
- 2 carrots, grated
- 1/4 red onion, thinly sliced
- 1/4 cup of apple cider vinegar
- 2 tbsp olive oil
- 1 tbsp honey or maple syrup
- 1 tsp Dijon mustard
- Salt and pepper to taste
- Optional: fresh herbs like parsley or cilantro, chopped

## Instructions

1. Combine the shredded cabbage, red cabbage, grated carrots and red onion in a large bowl.
2. Whisk apple cider vinegar with olive oil, honey or maple syrup (if using), Dijon mustard, salt and black pepper.
3. Douse the salad with dressing until well coated. Let it sit for a couple of minutes to blend flavors.
4. Garnish the coleslaw with an optional garnish of fresh herbs.

**Nutrition (Per Serving):**

Calories: 150 kcal Protein: 3 g Carbohydrates: 20 g Fats: 7 g Fiber: 4 g

# 3. Shrimp Taco Salad

**Prep Time: 15 minutes Cook Time: 10 minutes Servings: 4**

## Ingredients

- 500 grams of shrimp, peeled and deveined
- 1 tsp chili powder
- 1/2 tsp ground cumin
- 1/2 tsp garlic powder
- Salt and pepper to taste
- 2 tbsp olive oil
- 4 cups of mixed salad greens
- 1 cup of cherry tomatoes, halved
- 1 avocado, diced
- 1/2 cup of black beans, rinsed and drained
- 1/2 cup of corn kernels (fresh, canned, or thawed if frozen)
- 1/4 cup of red onion, finely chopped
- 1/4 cup of cilantro, chopped
- Juice of 1 lime
- Optional: grated cheese, sour cream, or salsa for topping

## Instructions

1. Throw the shrimp in a bowl with chili powder, cumin, garlic powder, salt and pepper.
2. Put some olive oil in a pan and heat it using medium heat. Put the shrimp on it and fry for 2-3 minutes on each side until they turn pink and cooked correctly.
3. Mix greens, cherry tomatoes, avocadoes, black beans, corn, and red onions with the cooked shrimp in one large bowl.
4. Sprinkle lime juice over the salad, tossing gently. Garnish with parsley. If desired, serve topped with optional accompaniments like grated cheese, sour cream or salsa.

**Nutrition (Per Serving):**

Calories: 300 kcal Protein: 30 g Carbohydrates: 25 g Fats: 15 g Fiber: 8 g

# 4. Italian Pasta Salad



## Ingredients

- 2 cups of whole wheat or whole grain pasta (such as penne or rotini)
- 1 cup of cherry tomatoes, halved
- 1/2 cup of black olives, sliced
- 1/2 cup of red onion, thinly sliced
- 1/2 cup of cucumber, diced
- 1/2 cup of bell pepper (any color), diced
- 1/4 cup of fresh basil leaves, chopped
- 1/4 cup of Parmesan cheese, grated
- 1/3 cup of Italian dressing
- Salt and pepper to taste

Optional: 1/4 cup of sun-dried tomatoes, chopped artichokes, or mozzarella cheese

## Instructions

1. Put the pasta in boiling water and cook as directed on the package until tender. Rinse them off with cold water and drain.
2. Combine the cooked pasta, cherry tomatoes, black olives, red onions, cucumbers, bell peppers, and fresh basil in a big bowl.
3. Pour Italian dressing over the salad; toss lightly to coat. Add grated Parmesan cheese; toss again.
4. Salt and pepper should be used for seasoning. To achieve the best taste possible, this salad should be chilled in a fridge for at least one hour before serving.
5. Serve pasta salad cold with optional ingredients if desired.

**Nutrition (Per Serving):**

Calories: 300 kcal Protein: 10 g Carbohydrates: 45 g Fats: 10 g Fiber: 8 g

# 5. Red Onion and Olive Focaccia

**Prep Time: 1 hour 20 minutes Cook Time: 20-25 minutes Servings: 8**

## Ingredients

- 500 grams of all-purpose flour
- 1 packet (7 grams) instant yeast
- 1 tsp sugar
- 1 1/2 tsp salt
- 300 ml warm water
- 1/4 cup of olive oil, plus extra for drizzling
- 1 large red onion, thinly sliced
- 1/2 cup of black olives, pitted and halved
- 2 tsp dried rosemary or fresh rosemary leaves

Sea salt flakes for sprinkling

## Instructions

1. Mix flour, yeast, sugar, and salt in a big bowl. Add warm water gradually and ¼ cup of olive oil while stirring to get a soft dough.
2. Place on a floured surface and knead until smooth for approximately 10 minutes.
3. Transfer the dough to a light-oiled bowl, cover it with a damp cloth and leave it in a warm place to rise for about an hour or until doubled.
4. Start preheating the oven to 200°C (400°F).
5. Knock back the dough and form it into a large, flat oval or rectangle on a baking sheet. Dimple with fingers. Sprinkle rosemary and sea salt flakes, drizzle more oil over the top, and scatter sliced red onion, followed by black olives.
6. Allow the dough to rise further for another 20 minutes.
7. Put in a preheated oven for 20-25 minutes or golden browned throughout when cooked.
8. Cool focaccia slightly before cutting it into pieces and serving it.

**Nutrition (Per Serving):**

Calories: 300 kcal Protein: 6 g Carbohydrates: 45-50 g Fats: 7 g Fiber: 2 g

# 6. Summer Squash Casserole

**Prep Time: 15 minutes Cook Time: 35 minutes Servings: 6**

## Ingredients

- 4 cups of summer squash (such as zucchini and yellow squash), sliced
- 1 large onion, chopped
- 2 garlic cloves, minced
- 1 cup of grated low-fat cheddar cheese
- 1/2 cup of whole wheat breadcrumbs
- 1/2 cup of low-fat milk
- 2 eggs, beaten
- 2 tbsp olive oil
- Salt and pepper to taste
- Optional: fresh herbs like basil or thyme, chopped

## Instructions

1. Put your oven to 180°C and grease a casserole pan lightly.
2. Sauté the chopped onion and minced garlic till they become soft. Add the sliced summer squash and cook until it is tender. Flavor with salt and pepper; add herbs if desired.
3. Mix the cooked vegetables with the beaten eggs, milk, and half of the cheese in a large bowl.
4. Empty the squash mixture into the greased casserole pan. Put breadcrumbs and the remaining cheese on top of that. Drizzle everything with olive oil.
5. The oven should bake everything for around 25-30 minutes until golden brown.
6. Serve when cooled only slightly.

**Nutrition Information (Per Serving):**

Calories: 220 kcal Protein: 12 g Carbohydrates: 20 g Fats: 10 g Fiber: 4 g

# 7. Roasted Butternut Squash

**Prep Time: 15 minutes Cook Time: 40 minutes Servings: 4**

## Ingredients

- 1 large butternut squash, peeled, seeded, and cut into 1-inch cubes
- 2 tbsp olive oil
- 1 tsp cinnamon
- 1/2 tsp nutmeg
- Salt and pepper to taste
- Optional: honey or maple syrup for a sweet glaze

## Instructions

1. Set your oven to 200°C (400°F).
2. Toss butternut squash cubes in a large bowl with olive oil, cinnamon, nutmeg, salt and pepper till well coated. For sweet glaze lovers, let that honey or maple syrup trickle on your squash.
3. Seasoned squash should be spread out onto a baking sheet as a single layer. They can then be roasted in the oven for about forty minutes until tender and lightly caramelized, turning halfway through cooking.
4. Take them out of the oven, and sprinkle some fresh herbs on top before serving.

**Nutrition (Per Serving):**

Calories: 180 kcal Protein: 2 g Carbohydrates: 30 g Fats: 9 g Fiber: 4 g

# 8. Stuffed Mushrooms

**Prep Time: 20 minutes Cook Time: 20 minutes Servings: 4**

## Ingredients

- 16 large button or cremini mushrooms, stems removed and chopped
- 1/4 cup of olive oil
- 2 cloves garlic, minced
- 1/2 cup of breadcrumbs
- 1/4 cup of grated Parmesan cheese
- 1/4 cup of chopped parsley
- Salt and pepper to taste

- Optional: 1/4 cup of finely chopped nuts or crumbled feta cheese for added texture and flavor

## Instructions

1. Set your oven to 180°C (350°F). Line a baking sheet with parchment paper.
2. Apply olive oil on the mushroom caps and put them on the baking sheet, hollow side up.
3. Put 2 tbsp of olive oil in a frying pan to heat. Add chopped stems of mushrooms and minced garlic, and stir-fry until soft.
4. After cooking the mushroom stems, mix them with breadcrumbs, parmesan cheese, parsley and nuts or feta cheese if desired. Add salt and pepper.
5. Gently push the filling into each cap of the mushroom firmly.
6. Bake for 20 minutes in an oven that has already been heated until mushrooms are tender and the tops have turned golden brown.
7. Serve warm.

**Nutrition (Per Serving):**

Calories: 200 kcal Protein: 5 g Carbohydrates: 15 g Fats: 10 g Fiber: 2 g

# 9. Italian Tuna Salad

**Prep Time: 15 minutes Cook Time: 0 minutes Servings: 4**

## Ingredients

- 2 cans of tuna in olive oil, drained
- 1 cup of cherry tomatoes, halved
- 1/2 cup of black olives, pitted and sliced
- 1/4 cup of red onion, thinly sliced
- 1/4 cup of fresh basil leaves, torn
- 2 tbsp capers, drained
- Juice of 1 lemon
- 3 tbsp extra virgin olive oil
- Salt and pepper to taste

Optional: 1/4 cup of shaved Parmesan cheese or a handful of arugula leaves

## Instructions

1. Take one big bowl and then mix it up with the drained tuna, cherry tomatoes, black olives, red onions, basil leaves and capers.
2. Using a small bowl, mix lemon juice, olive oil, extra virgin salt, and pepper.
3. The dressing should then be put on the salad before being gently tossed.
4. You may garnish the salad with shaved Parmesan cheese or sprinkle a handful of arugula leaves for added flavor and texture before serving.

**Nutrition (Per Serving):**

Calories: 250 kcal Protein: 20 g Carbohydrates: 10 g Fats: 15 g Fiber: 2 g

# 10. Avocado and Tuna Salad

**Prep Time: 10 minutes Cook Time: 0 minutes Servings: 2-3**

## Ingredients

- 2 cans of tuna in water, drained
- 2 ripe avocados, peeled, pitted, and diced
- 1/2 red onion, finely chopped
- 1/2 red bell pepper, diced
- 1/4 cup of fresh cilantro (or parsley), chopped
- Juice of 1 lime
- 2 tbsp olive oil
- Salt and pepper to taste

Optional: 1 tbsp of mayonnaise or Greek yogurt for creaminess

## Instructions

1. Mix the cut avocados, drained tunas, chopped onions, and parsley or cilantro in a large bowl.
2. If desired, combine lime juice, olive oil, and perhaps mayonnaise or Greek yogurt in a small bowl. Spice with salt as well as pepper.
3. Pour the dressing over the tuna avocado mixture; mix gently until they are well blended, and the avocado is coated to stop browning.
4. Serve immediately or refrigerate for about an hour before serving so that all tastes can blend.

**Nutrition (Per Serving)**

Calories: 350 kcal Protein: 25 g Carbohydrates: 15 g Fats: 25 g Fiber: 10 g

# 11. Garlic Parmesan Fries

**Prep Time: 15 minutes Cook Time: 30 minutes Servings: 4**

## Ingredients

- 4 large potatoes, peeled and cut into fry-shaped sticks
- 4 tbsp olive oil
- 3 cloves garlic, minced
- 1/2 cup of grated Parmesan cheese
- 1 tbsp fresh parsley, chopped
- Salt and pepper to taste

## Instructions

1. Set your oven to 220°C (425°F). Line a baking sheet with parchment paper.
2. Soak the fries in cold water for at least 30 minutes. This step helps remove excess starch and makes the fries crispy.
3. Drain your potatoes thoroughly and dry them with a towel. Then, season with olive oil (3 tbsp), salt, and pepper.
4. Lay out the French fries on the baking sheet so that they are in one layer. Bake in preheated oven for about 30 minutes, turning halfway through, until golden brown and crispy.
5. While the fries are baking, heat the olive oil in a small frying pan over medium-high heat; add minced garlic clove until fragrant. Remove from heat and mix in grated Parmesan cheese & chopped parsley.
6. Finally, when your fries are ready, toss them with the garlic-Parmesan mixture while they're still hot.
7. Serve immediately.

**Nutrition (Per Serving)**

Calories: 350 kcal Protein: 6 g Carbohydrates: 45 g Fats: 18 g Fiber: 4 g

# 12. Cilantro Lime Low-Carb Rice

**Prep Time: 10 minutes Cook Time: 10 minutes Servings: 4**

## Ingredients

- 1 large cauliflower head
- 2 tbsp olive oil
- Juice and zest of 1 lime
- 1/4 cup of fresh cilantro, chopped
- Salt and pepper to taste
- Optional: 1 garlic clove, minced, or red pepper flakes for a spicy kick

## Instructions

1. To remove the stems and leaves, chop a cauliflower into chunks. You can also blend the cauliflower in a food processor until it looks like rice or use a box grater to grate it.
2. In a large skillet, heat olive oil over medium heat. Cook the cauliflower rice for about 5-7 minutes or until cooked but slightly firm.
3. Take away the skillet from the heat. Add in lime juice and zest, as well as chopped cilantro. Adjust to taste with pepper and salt.
4. Serve hot as a side dish with cilantro lime cauliflower rice.

**Nutrition (Per Serving):**

Calories: 120 kcal Protein: 4 g Carbohydrates: 12 g Fats: 7 g Fiber: 5 g

# 13. Citrus Spinach



## Ingredients

- 4 cups of fresh spinach leaves
- 1 orange, segmented
- 1 lemon, zested and juiced
- 2 tbsp olive oil
- 2 cloves garlic, minced
- Salt and pepper to taste

Optional: 1/4 cup of slivered almonds or chopped walnuts for crunch

## Instructions

1. Wash the spinach leaves entirely and dry them.
2. Heat the olive oil in a big skillet over medium heat. Put the ground garlic in and cook for about 1 minute to make it fragrant but not browned.
3. Put the spinach into your pan. Stir often until it begins to wilt, about 2-3 minutes. Be careful not to let it cook more than necessary, as it should still be somewhat crunchy when done.
4. Remove from the stove after cooking. Add orange segments, lemon zest and juice that you have just squeezed onto spinach in a skillet, then mix gently.
5. Add salt and pepper according to taste. Add slivered almonds or chopped walnuts on top for extra crunchiness if desired. Serve at once.

**Nutrition (Per Serving):**

Calories: 100 kcal Protein: 3 g Carbohydrates: 10 g Fats: 5 g Fiber: 3 g

# 14. Vegetarian Cakes

**Prep Time: 20 minutes Cook Time: 15 minutes Servings: 4**

## Ingredients

- 2 cups of cooked quinoa or mixed grains
- 1 cup of canned chickpeas, drained and rinsed
- 1/2 cup of breadcrumbs
- 1/2 cup of grated carrot
- 1/2 cup of finely chopped bell peppers
- 1/4 cup of finely chopped onion
- 1/4 cup of chopped fresh parsley or cilantro
- 2 cloves garlic, minced
- 2 large eggs, beaten
- 1 tsp paprika
- 1/2 tsp cumin
- Salt and pepper to taste
- 2-3 tbsp olive oil for frying

Optional: Greek yogurt or a light sour cream for serving

## Instructions

1. In a big bowl, squash the chickpeas lightly. Add cooked quinoa, breadcrumbs, grated carrot, bell peppers, onion, parsley or cilantro, minced garlic, beaten eggs, paprika, cumin powder, salt and pepper. Mix until the ingredients are well blended.
2. Divide the mixture and shape it into eight flat round cakes.
3. Place olive oil in a large nonstick skillet set over medium heat. Cook the cakes on each side for about 3-4 minutes in batches until golden brown and crispy.
4. Optionally serve hot with Greek yogurt or light sour cream atop vegetarian cakes.

**Nutrition (Per Serving)**

Calories: 250 kcal Protein: 8 g Carbohydrates: 35 g Fats: 7 g Fiber: 6 g

# 15. Curried Chickpea Salad



## Ingredients

- 2 cans (about 400 grams each) of chickpeas, rinsed and drained
- 1/2 cup of plain Greek yogurt (low-fat)
- 1 tbsp curry powder
- 1 tsp ground cumin
- 1 small red onion, finely chopped
- 1 red bell pepper, diced
- 1/2 cup of raisins or chopped dried apricots
- 1/4 cup of chopped fresh cilantro
- Salt and pepper to taste

Optional: 1/4 cup of chopped almonds or cashews for added crunch

## Instructions

1. Combine chickpeas, red onions, bell peppers, raisins, dry apricots, and coriander in a big bowl.
2. Curry powder and cumin mixed with Greek yoghurt can be poured into another bowl. Salt and pepper to taste.
3. Pour the mix of these ingredients on the chickpea; stir them well until they look combined properly. Allow it to stay in the refrigerator for at least 30 minutes before you serve it so that flavors can blend.
4. To add more texture and flavor to the salad, chop some nuts on top before serving.

**Nutrition (Per Serving)**

Calories: 300 kcal Protein: 10g Carbohydrates: 50 g Fats: 5 g Fiber: 12 g

# 16. Lentil and Feta Tabbouleh

**Prep Time: 20 minutes Cook Time: 20 minutes Servings: 4**

## Ingredients

- 1 cup of dried green or brown lentils
- 1 cup of bulgur wheat
- 2 cups of boiling water
- 1 cucumber, diced
- 2 medium tomatoes, diced
- 1/2 cup of red onion, finely chopped
- 1/2 cup of fresh parsley, chopped
- 1/4 cup of fresh mint, chopped
- 1/3 cup of feta cheese, crumbled
- 1/4 cup of olive oil
- Juice of 2 lemons
- Salt and pepper to taste

Optional: 1 tbsp pomegranate molasses or a handful of pomegranate seeds

## Instructions

1. Place the lentils under a running tap and put them in hot water for boiling, which will take about 20 minutes to be ready. After this, they should be drained and cooled.
2. Get one big bowl where you can put bulgur before pouring two cups of boiling water. Allow it to sit for 10-15 minutes until it absorbs the water and becomes tender. Use a fork to separate it into separate little grains.
3. Put the bulgur in a large bowl with the cucumbers, feta cheese, mint, onion, tomatoes, red onion, cooked lentils, and parsley.
4. Combine olive oil with lemon juice; add salt and pepper. This dressing must be poured on tabbouleh and mixed thoroughly until all flavors are absorbed into the meal.
5. The tabbouleh must stay in the fridge for at least an hour so that its flavor will mix well together. You may also add pomegranate molasses over it or sprinkle pomegranate seeds on top as desired.

**Nutrition (Per Serving)**

Calories: 350 kcal Protein: 15 g Carbohydrates: 45 g Fats: 15 g Fiber: 12 g

# 17. Garlic Mashed Sweet Potatoes

**Prep Time: 10 minutes Cook Time: 30 minutes Servings: 4**

## Ingredients

- 4 large sweet potatoes, peeled and cubed
- 3 cloves of garlic, minced
- 1/4 cup of low-fat milk or almond milk
- 2 tbsp unsalted butter or olive oil
- Salt and pepper to taste
- Optional: Fresh herbs like thyme or rosemary, chopped

## Instructions

1. Take the cubed sweet potatoes and boil them in salted water. Bring to a boil and cook until tender, about 20-25 minutes.
2. While boiling the sweet potatoes, fry the minced garlic in a tiny saucepan with a bit of butter or olive oil to get fragrant, approximately 1-2 minutes. Make sure not to overcook.
3. Drain the cooked sweet potatoes and return them to the pot. Add sautéed garlic, milk, butter or olive oil, plus some salt and pepper to taste in there. Mash well till smooth and creamy. Adjust seasoning.
4. Serve hot mashed sweet potatoes topped with optional fresh herbs.

**Nutrition (Per Serving):**

Calories: -250 kcal Protein: 3-g Carbohydrates: 35-40 g Fats: 5-7 g Fiber: 5-6 g Sodium: Low

# CHAPTER 6: DESSERTS

## 1. Cinnamon Protein Apple Slices

**Prep Time: 10 minutes Cook Time: 0 minutes Servings: 2**

## Ingredients

- 2 large apples, cored and sliced
- 1/2 cup of Greek yogurt
- 2 tbsp almond butter or peanut butter
- 1 scoop vanilla or plain protein powder
- 1 tsp cinnamon

Optional toppings: Chopped nuts, a drizzle of honey, or a sprinkle of granola

## Instructions

1. You can wash the apples, cut them into rounds or wedges, and remove the cores.
2. Mix Greek yoghurt with either almond butter or peanut butter in a bowl until it is well mixed; add protein powder and mix well. Mix in cinnamon to make the mixture smooth.
3. Apply a layer of protein mixture on each slice of apple.
4. To give some texture and taste, sprinkle optional toppings on apple slices.
5. Serve the cinnamon protein apple slices right away like a healthy snack after dinner.

**Nutrition (Per Serving)**

Calories: 220 kcal Protein: 10 g Carbohydrates: 25 g Fats: 6 g Fiber: 5 g

# 2. Triple Berry Yogurt Parfait

**Prep Time: 10 minutes Cook Time: 0 minutes Servings: 4**

## Ingredients

- 2 cups of Greek yogurt
- 1 cup of fresh strawberries, sliced
- 1 cup of fresh blueberries
- 1 cup of fresh raspberries
- 1/4 cup of granola
- 2 tbsp honey or maple syrup (optional)
- Optional: a few mint leaves for garnish

## Instructions

1. Place some Greek yoghurt at the bottom of four glasses or parfait cups.
2. Put a layer of mixed berries (strawberries, blueberries, raspberries) on top of the yogurt.
3. Keep adding yogurt and berries in layers until the glass is nearly complete. Depending on the size of your glasses or cups, you can pile them in as many layers as you want.
4. Scatter granola over the last layer of berries.
5. If someone wants more sweetness, they can add honey or maple syrup to the granola.
6. End it with mint leaves. The parfait should be served right away; otherwise, place it in the refrigerator for up to 30 minutes before serving.

**Nutrition (Per Serving):**

Calories: 200 kcal Protein: 12 g Carbohydrates: 25 g Fats: 4 g Fiber: 4 g Sodium: Low

# 3. Frozen Chocolate Banana

**Prep Time: 15 minute Cook Time: 0 minutes Servings: 4**

## Ingredients

- 4 ripe bananas
- 200 grams of dark chocolate
- 1 tbsp coconut oil

Optional toppings: chopped nuts, shredded coconut, sprinkles, or sea salt

## Instructions

1. Peel off the bananas and reduce them into halves horizontally. Into every half, stick iced popsicles and lay them on a baking sheet covered with wax paper, then allow them to freeze completely for about two hours.
2. Disintegrate dark chocolate into smaller pieces and melt it with coconut oil in a microwave-safe bowl. Continually stir this mixture until the chocolate is entirely melted and smooth.
3. The melted chocolate should be placed in a large bowl just after dipping these frozen bananas so that the chocolate leaves no side uncoated. You can allow any excess drip off.
4. Whichever additional toppings you choose should be spread over the bananas before they set
5. Put back your parchment paper when you are done freezing your chocolates to have them set, which might take around fifteen minutes.
6. Eat right away or store in a sealed container or freezer bag.

**Nutrition (Per Serving):**

Calories: 300 kcal Protein: 3 g Carbohydrates: 35 g Fats: 10 g Fiber: 5 g Sodium: Low

# 4. Protein Sludge

**Prep Time: 5 minutes Cook Time: 0 minutes Servings: 1**

## Ingredients

- 1 scoop of protein powder
- 2 tbsp natural peanut butter or almond butter
- 1/2 cup of Greek yogurt
- 1 tbsp cocoa powder
- 1-2 tbsp milk or water

Optional toppings: sliced banana, berries, chia seeds, or a drizzle of honey

## Instructions

1. Put protein powder, peanut butter or almond butter, Greek yogurt and cocoa powder in a bowl.
2. Slowly pour milk or water into the mixture and keep stirring until it becomes thick, like sludge.
3. You can add toppings such as sliced bananas, berries, chia seeds or honey dripping on top of it to make it more flavored and nutritious. Enjoy.

**Nutrition (Per Serving):**

Calories: 350 kcal Protein: 25 g Carbohydrates: 15 g Fats: 20 g Fiber: 4 g

# 5. Apple Crisp

**Prep Time: 15 minutes Cook Time: 45 minutes Servings: 6**

## Ingredients

- 5-6 medium apples, peeled, cored, and sliced
- 1/2 cup of granulated sugar
- 1 tsp ground cinnamon
- 1/2 tsp nutmeg
- 1 cup of old-fashioned oats
- 1/2 cup of whole wheat flour
- 1/2 cup of brown sugar
- 1/2 cup of unsalted butter, cold and cut into small pieces

- Optional: 1/2 cup of chopped walnuts or pecans

## Instructions

1. Set your oven to 180°C (350°F). Grease a 9-inch baking pan.
2. Stir the apple slices with granulated sugar, cinnamon, and nutmeg in a bowl. Spread out the apple mixture prepared gently on the baking pan.
3. Mix oats, whole wheat flour, and brown sugar in another bowl. Include cold butter pieces, and with your fingertips or pastry cutter, work the butter into the oat mixture until it resembles coarse crumbs. Add nuts if using.
4. The oat mixture is then sprinkled evenly over the apples.
5. Preheat oven and bake for about 45 minutes or till the topping is golden brown and the apples are tender.
6. When you're done, cool it out of the oven before serving. It may be served warm or at room temperature.

**Nutrition (Per Serving):**

Calories: 350 kcal Protein: 3 g Carbohydrates: 55 g Fats: 15 g Fiber: 5 g

# 6. Paleo Brownies

**Prep Time: 15 minutes Cook Time: 25 minutes Servings: 8-10**

## Ingredients

- 1 cup of almond flour
- 1/4 cup of cocoa powder
- 1/2 tsp baking soda
- 1/4 tsp salt
- 1/2 cup of honey or pure maple syrup
- 1/3 cup of coconut oil, melted
- 2 large eggs
- 1 tsp vanilla extract
- Optional: 1/2 cup of dark chocolate chips

## Instructions

1. Set your oven to 175°C (350°F). Line an 8-inch square baking pan with parchment paper.
2. Take the almond flour, cocoa powder, baking soda and salt to a large bowl and whisk.

3.  Add honey (or maple syrup), melted coconut oil, eggs, and vanilla extract to another bowl and mix well.
4.  Combine both dry ingredients with wet ones by pouring in small amounts. If there's any need for chocolate chips, include them as well.
5.  Carefully pour this batter into the prepared pan, ensuring it is spread uniformly. Bake for 20-25 minutes or until a toothpick inserted near the center comes out clean.
6.  Cut the brownies into squares after they have cooled down in the pan.

**Nutrition (Per Serving):**

Calories: 250 kcal Protein: 4 g Carbohydrates: 20 g Fats: 16 g Fiber: 3 g

# 7. Keto Cheesecake

**Prep Time: 20 minutes Cook Time: 50 minutes Servings: 10**

## Ingredients

For the Crust:

- 1 1/2 cups of almond flour
- 1/4 cup of butter, melted
- 1 tbsp erythritol
- 1/2 tsp vanilla extract

For the Filling:

- 24 ounces cream cheese, softened
- 1 cup of erythritol
- 3 large eggs
- 1 tbsp lemon juice
- 1 tsp vanilla extract

## Instructions

1.  Set your oven to 160°C (325°F).
2.  Combine this with melted butter, erythritol, and vanilla extract in a bowl. This mixture must be pressed into the bottom of a 9-inch spring form pan to form an even crust. Take it out and cool it after 10 minutes of baking time.
3.  Mix cream cheese and erythritol until smooth. Incorporate eggs one at a time, ensuring each is thoroughly blended before adding another. Stir in lemon juice and vanilla extract.

4. Spread the cream cheese filling over the cooled crust using a spatula to smoothen the top.
5. Bake for 40-50 minutes or until set but still slightly jiggly in the center of the cheesecake. Turn off the oven; let the cheesecake sit in the oven with the door closed for 1 hour.
6. Remove from the oven and allow it to cool to room temperature, then refrigerate for at least four hours or overnight if possible.
7. Serve cold by slicing.

**Nutrition (Per Serving):**

Calories: 350 kcal Protein: 7 g Carbohydrates: 5g Fats: 30 g Fiber: 2 g

# 8. Frozen Banana Yogurt Bark

**Prep Time: 10 minutes Freezing Time: 4 hours Servings: 6**

## Ingredients

- 2 cups of Greek yogurt
- 2 ripe bananas, mashed
- 2 tbsp honey or maple syrup (optional)
- 1/2 cup of mixed berries
- 1/4 cup of granola
- 1/4 cup of chopped nuts

Optional: a sprinkle of shredded coconut, dark chocolate chips, or chia seeds

## Instructions

1. Mix the Greek yogurt, mashed bananas, honey, or maple syrup in a bowl.
2. Cover the baking sheet or large tray with parchment paper.
3. Empty the yogurt mixture onto the lined baking sheet and smoothen it out evenly.
4. Distribute mixed berries, granola or chopped nuts over the yoghurt. Add coconut, chocolate chips, chia seeds, or other toppings for more flavors.
5. Place it into the freezer until it becomes hard enough to cut into 4 hours approx. Keep it in the freezer for about six hours, but overnight is still better for solidifying the mixture into ice cubes, which must be separated only later.
6. Once that is done, break apart or cut up your frozen yogurt bark.
7. Serve immediately as a frozen treat.

Calories: 200 kcal Protein: 10 g Carbohydrates: 25 g Fats: 4 g Fiber: 3 g

# 9. No-Bake Cookie Bites

**Prep Time: 15 minutes Chilling Time: 30 minutes Servings: 12-15 bites**

## Ingredients

- 1 cup of rolled oats
- 1/2 cup of natural peanut butter or almond butter
- 1/3 cup of honey or maple syrup
- 1/2 cup of ground flaxseed
- 1/4 cup of mini dark chocolate chips
- 1 tsp vanilla extract
- A pinch of salt

Optional: 2 tbsp chia seeds or protein powder for added nutrition

## Instructions

1. Combine oats, peanut butter or almond butter, honey or maple syrup, ground flaxseed, mini chocolate chips, vanilla extract, and salt in a large bowl. Chia seeds or protein powder can be added if desired.
2. Form small balls about 1 inch in diameter by rolling the mixture with your hands. Set them on a baking sheet or tray covered with parchment paper.
3. Put the bites in the fridge for at least half an hour to harden.
4. Take these no-bake cookie bites right out of the refrigerator. Leftovers can be stored inside an airtight container in the fridge.

**Nutrition (Per Bite):**

Calories: 140 kcal Protein: 4 g Carbohydrates: 18 g Fats: 7 g Fiber: 3 g

# 10. Almond Cookies

**Prep Time: 15 minutes Cook Time: 12 minutes Servings: 12 cookies**

## Ingredients

- 2 cups of almond flour
- 1/2 cup of granulated sugar
- 1/4 cup of unsalted butter, softened
- 1 large egg
- 1 tsp vanilla extract
- 1/2 tsp baking powder
- A pinch of salt
- Optional: 1/4 cup of sliced almonds for topping

## Instructions

1. Set your oven to 175°C (350°F). Line a baking sheet with parchment paper.
2. Whisk the almond flour, sugar (or sugar substitute), baking powder, and salt in a bowl.
3. Soften the butter, egg and vanilla extract to the dry components. Mix them until they form a dough.
4. Form balls from small portions of dough. Place on the prepared baking sheet and flatten gently with your palm or the back of a spoon. If you want, press some sliced almonds on each cookie.
5. Bake 10-12 minutes in a preheated oven until the edges turn brown.
6. Cool them on the sheet for a few minutes, then shift to a wire rack for complete cooling.

**Nutrition (Per Cookie):**

Calories: 170 kcal Protein: 5 g Carbohydrates: 12 g Fats: 14 g Fiber: 3 g Sodium: Low

# 11. Apple Oatmeal Crunchy

**Prep Time: 20 minutes Cook Time: 30-35 minutes Servings: 6**

## Ingredients

- 3 large apples, peeled, cored, and sliced
- 1 cup of rolled oats
- 1/2 cup of whole wheat flour
- 1/2 cup of brown sugar or a brown sugar substitute
- 1/2 cup of unsalted butter, melted
- 1 tsp ground cinnamon
- 1/2 tsp nutmeg
- A pinch of salt

Optional: 1/4 cup of chopped walnuts or almonds for added texture

## Instructions

1. Set your oven at 180°C (350°F). Grease an 8-inch square baking pan.
2. The sliced apples should be arranged at the bottom of the baking pan. Sprinkle with half a tsp of cinnamon and nutmeg.
3. In a bowl, combine rolled oats, whole wheat flour, brown sugar or sugars you use instead, remaining cinnamon & nutmeg and also a pinch of salt. Melt the butter, then tip it into the oat mixture. Use your fingertips to mix until coarse crumbs form. Add nuts if you want to.
4. Finally, sprinkle this oat mixture evenly over the apples in the pan.
5. Place in oven and bake for about 30 – 35 minutes or until golden brown topping is seen on top and apples are tender when pierced with a fork.
6. Allow to cool slightly before serving; serve warm or at room temperature.

**Nutrition (Per Serving):**

Calories: 300 kcal Protein: 4 g Carbohydrates: 45 g Fats: 15 g Fiber: 4 g Sodium: Low

# 12. Chocolate Banana Cups

**Prep Time: 15 minutes Freezing Time: 2 hours Servings: 12 cups**

## Ingredients

- 2 large bananas, ripe but firm
- 1 cup of dark chocolate chips
- 1 tbsp coconut oil

Optional toppings: sea salt flakes, shredded coconut, or chopped nuts

## Instructions

1. Line a mini muffin tin with paper liners, or use a silicone mold to hold the paper cups in place.
2. Put chocolate chips and coconut oil in a microwavable bowl. Depending on the size of the chips, microwave for 30 seconds at a time until the chocolate is smooth.
3. Place some of the melted chocolate into each cup. Cut bananas into rounds about 1/2 inch thick; put one piece in per cup. If fillings are being used, then add a little bit more banana on top of it all. After covering all the banana cuts with even more melted chocolate to be fully wrapped, remember to sprinkle them with optional toppings like sea salt, coconut or nuts.
4. Freeze these cups for 2 hours or until firm.
5. When frozen, remove from pans to serve immediately or keep in freezer in an airtight container.

**Nutrition (Per Cup):**

Calories: 120 kcal Protein: 2 g Carbohydrates: 15 g Fats: 6 g Fiber: 2 g Sodium: Low

# 13. Apple Pie Bars

**Prep Time: 20 minutes Cook Time: 45 minutes Servings: 12 bars**

## Ingredients

For the Crust and Topping:

- 2 1/2 cups of all-purpose flour
- 1 cup of unsalted butter, cold and cubed
- 1/2 cup of granulated sugar
- 1/2 tsp salt

For the Apple Filling:

- 4 large apples, peeled, cored, and thinly sliced
- 2 tbsp granulated sugar
- 1 tsp ground cinnamon
- 1/4 tsp ground nutmeg
- 1 tbsp all-purpose flour

## Instructions

1. To bake, heat your oven at 180°C (350°F) and line a 9x13 inch baking pan with parchment paper to make it easier to remove the baked goods.
2. Mix flour, sugar, and salt in a large bowl. Add the cold butter with your hands or a pastry cutter until the mixture resembles crumbs. One cup of this prepared mix is reserved while the rest is pressed into the bottom of the prepared baking pan.
3. Remove from oven after 15 minutes.
4. Combine sliced apples with sugar (2 tbsp.), cinnamon, nutmeg and flour (1 tbsp.). Put apple slices over the crust that has already been baked.
5. The apple-filled crust should now be topped with a sprinkling of crumbs you had set aside.
6. Bake for 30-35 minutes until the top slightly turns golden brown.
7. When cool, remove bars from the pan using parchment paper as handles and cut them into squares.

**Nutrition (Per Bar):**

Calories: 300 kcal Protein: 2 g Carbohydrates: 40 g Fats: 12 g Fiber: 2 g Sodium: Low

# 14. Cinnamon Apple Protein Bars



## Ingredients

- 2 cups of rolled oats
- 1/2 cup of vanilla protein powder
- 1 tsp cinnamon
- 1/2 tsp nutmeg
- 1/4 tsp salt
- 1 cup of unsweetened applesauce
- 1/4 cup of honey or maple syrup
- 1/4 cup of almond milk
- 1 apple, peeled and finely chopped
- Optional: 1/4 cup of chopped nuts or raisins

## Instructions

1. Set your oven to 180°C (350°F). Line an 8-inch square baking pan with parchment paper.
2. Mix the protein powder, nutmeg, salt, cinnamon and rolled oats in a large bowl.
3. Then stir in almond milk, honey or maple syrup, and unsweetened applesauce. Mix well.
4. Mix thoroughly until you distribute the chopped apple and other things, such as nuts or raisins, into it.
5. Spread this with a spatula across the prepared baking pan and then bake for 18-20 minutes until the edges turn brownish and the center solidifies.
6. When done baking for about twenty to twenty-five minutes at three sixty degrees Fahrenheit, as explained above, take them out of the oven.
7. When cool, lift them out with parchment paper after an hour. Cut into twelve bars.

**Nutrition (Per Bar):**

Calories: 170 kcal Protein: 9 g Carbohydrates: 30 g Fats: 4 g Fiber: 4 g Sodium: Low

# 15. Peanut Butter Protein Cookies

**Prep Time: 10 minutes Cook Time: 10-12 minutes Servings: 12 cookies**

## Ingredients

- 1 cup of natural peanut butter
- 1/3 cup of protein powder
- 1/4 cup of honey or maple syrup
- 1 large egg
- 1 tsp vanilla extract
- 1/2 tsp baking soda
- A pinch of salt
- Optional: dark chocolate chips or chopped nuts for added texture

## Instructions

1. Set your oven to 180°C (350°F). Line a baking sheet with parchment paper.
2. The peanut butter, protein powder, honey or maple syrup, egg, vanilla extract, soda and salt are mixed in a mixer to form a smooth blend. Ensure that all the ingredients are well blended. Otherwise, chocolate chips or nuts may be added.
3. Take a tbsp of the dough and shape it into balls. Then, press gently with a fork on top to get crisscross marks on the cookies.
4. Bake at 350°F for 10-12 minutes until edges turn light golden brown.
5. Leave cookies on the baking sheet for a few minutes before transferring them to a wire rack to cool completely.

**Nutrition (Per Cookie):**

Calories: 200 kcal Protein: 9 g Carbohydrates: 15 g Fats: 12 g Fiber: 3 g Sodium: Low

# 16. Café Mocha Protein Bars

**Prep Time: 15 minutes Chilling Time: 1 hour Servings: 12 bars**

## Ingredients

- 1 cup of rolled oats
- 1/2 cup of protein powder
- 1/4 cup of unsweetened cocoa powder
- 1/4 cup of strong brewed coffee, cooled
- 1/2 cup of almond butter or peanut butter
- 1/4 cup of honey or maple syrup
- 1 tsp vanilla extract

Optional: 1/4 cup of dark chocolate chips or cacao nibs for extra flavor

## Instructions

1. Mix the oats, protein powder, and cocoa in a big bowl.
2. Combine coffee, almond or peanut butter, honey or maple syrup and vanilla extract in another container.
3. Add wet ingredients to the dry ones until sticky dough forms. Add chocolate chips if using.
4. Cover an 8x8 inch baking pan with parchment paper and press the mixture into the pan firmly and evenly.
5. Refrigerate the bars for a minimum of one hour to allow them to be set completely.
6. Remove from pan after setting, then cut into 10-12 even pieces
7. Keep the bars in an airtight container in the fridge for up to one week.

**Nutrition (Per Bar)**

Calories: 200 kcal Protein: 10 g Carbohydrates: 20 g Fats: 9 g Fiber: 3 g Sodium: Low

# 17. High-Protein Oatmeal Cookies

**Prep Time: 15 minutes Cook Time: 10 minutes Servings: 12 cookies**

## Ingredients

- 2 cups of rolled oats
- 1/2 cup of protein powder
- 1/2 cup of almond butter or peanut butter
- 1/4 cup of honey or maple syrup
- 2 large eggs
- 1 tsp vanilla extract
- 1/2 tsp baking soda
- 1/2 tsp cinnamon
- A pinch of salt

Optional: 1/4 cup of dark chocolate chips or dried fruits (like raisins or cranberries)

## Instructions

1. Set your oven to 180°C (350°F). Line a baking sheet with parchment paper.
2. Combine the oatmeal, protein powder, baking soda, cinnamon, and salt in a big bowl.
3. Mix in almond butter (or peanut butter), honey (or maple syrup), eggs and vanilla extract to the dry ingredients. Mix well. If preferred, chocolate chips or dried fruits can be added.
4. Using a tablespoon, scoop dough onto an already prepared cookie sheet. Use your hand or a fork to flatten each cookie slightly.
5. Place into the preheated oven for about 10-12 minutes until you see the edges turn golden brown completely.
6. Cookies should cool on a baking sheet for some moments before being transferred onto wire racks, where they will be cooled entirely.

**Nutrition (Per Cookie):**

Calories: 180 kcal Protein: 6 g Carbohydrates: 18 g Fats: 9 g Fiber: 3 g Sodium: Low

# 18. Greek Yogurt Parfait

**Prep Time: 10 minutes Cook Time: 0 minutes Servings: 4**

## Ingredients

- 2 cups of Greek yogurt
- 1 cup of granola
- 1 cup of mixed berries
- 2 tbsp honey or maple syrup (optional)
- Optional toppings: nuts, seeds, or a sprinkle of cinnamon

## Instructions

1. Add scoops of Greek yogurt at the base in individual glasses or bowls.
2. After using the yoghurt, sprinkle granola and then mixed fruits.
3. Layer back and forth yogurt, granola and berries until they fill the glass. You can have as many layers as possible depending on your glasses' size
4. They may be sweetened with honey or maple syrup if desired. Alternatively, a little cinnamon seeds or nuts can be sprinkled on top.
5. The best texture will be found in a freshly made parfait; otherwise, it could be kept in the refrigerator for about one hour before serving it.

**Nutrition (Per Serving)**

Calories: 250 kcal Protein: 10 g Carbohydrates: 30 g Fats: 10 g Fiber: 4 g

# 19. Vegan Chocolate Chip Cookies

**Prep Time: 15 minutes Cook Time: 15 minutes Servings: 20 cookies**

## Ingredients

- 2 cups of all-purpose flour
- 1 tsp baking soda
- 1/2 tsp salt
- 1/2 cup of coconut oil, solid (not melted)
- 1/2 cup of brown sugar
- 1/2 cup of granulated sugar
- 1/4 cup of almond milk
- 2 tsp vanilla extract
- 1 cup of vegan chocolate chips

## Instructions

1. Set your oven to 180°C (350°F). Line a baking sheet with parchment paper.
2. Flour, baking soda and salt should be whisked together in a bowl.
3. In another large bowl, combine the brown sugar and granulated sugar with the solid coconut oil by beating them until you have a creamy mixture.
4. Mix almond milk and vanilla extract into the sugar mix.
5. Gradually add wet ingredients to dry ones and stir until dough is formed; fold in vegan chocolate chips.
6. Drop tablespoon of dough onto the prepared baking sheet about 2 inches apart, slightly flattening each one.
7. Place it into the preheated oven for around 12-15 minutes until the edges become golden-brownish.
8. Leave the cookies on the baking sheet to cool for some minutes before transferring them to wire racks, where they will completely cool down.

**Nutrition (Per Cookie):**

Calories: 170 kcal Protein: 3 g Carbohydrates: 22 g Fats: 9 g Fiber: 2 g Sodium: Low

# 20. Strawberry Shortcake

**Prep Time: 30 minutes Cook Time: 15-20 minutes Servings: 8**

## Ingredients

For the Shortcakes:

- 2 cups of all-purpose flour
- 1/4 cup of granulated sugar
- 1 tbsp baking powder
- 1/2 tsp salt
- 1/2 cup of unsalted butter, cold and cubed
- 2/3 cup of whole milk or cream
- 1 tsp vanilla extract

For the Topping:

- 2 cups of fresh strawberries, hulled and sliced
- 2 tbsp granulated sugar
- 1 cup of heavy whipping cream
- 1 tbsp powdered sugar
- 1/2 tsp vanilla extract

## Instructions

1. Set your oven to 200°C (400°F). Line a baking sheet with parchment paper.
2. Mix flour with 1/4 cup of granulated sugar, baking powder, and salt in a big bowl. Slice the cold butter into coarse crumbs using a pastry blender or your hands. Stir milk and vanilla extract in it until just moistened.
3. A medium-sized spoon drops dough on the prepared cookie sheet, lining them into 8 equal portions. Bake for 15-20 minutes until golden brown. Take it off the oven and let it cool on a rack.
4. Put sliced strawberries in another bowl and toss them with 2 tablespoon of granulated sugar. Set aside for about twenty minutes to macerate.
5. Whip the heavy whipping cream with powdered sugar and ½ tsp of vanilla extract in another bowl until stiff peaks are formed.
6. Split each shortcake horizontally. Spread some of the macerated strawberries over the bottom half of each biscuit, top with whipped cream, followed by the other half of the biscuit. Sprinkle more strawberries on top, and then end up with whipped cream.

# 1. Peanut Butter & Banana Smoothie

**Prep Time: 5 minutes Cook Time: 0 minutes Servings: 2**

## Ingredients

- 2 ripe bananas, peeled and sliced
- 2 tbsp natural peanut butter
- 1 cup of almond milk
- 1/2 cup of Greek yogurt
- 1 tbsp honey or maple syrup (optional)
- 1/2 tsp vanilla extract (optional)
- A handful of ice cubes

## Instructions

1. Put the bananas, peanut butter, almond milk, Greek yogurt, maple syrup or honey, vanilla extract and ice cubes into a blender.
2. Blend until smooth and creamy on high speed. If the consistency of the drink is thick, then you can add more of the milk to get it to where you want it.
3. Serve immediately to taste better and not lose its original texture as it cools down.

**Nutrition (Per Serving):**

Calories: 300 kcal Protein: 10 g Carbohydrates: 40 g Fats: 12 g Fiber: 4 g

# 2. Oatmeal & Berry Smoothie

**Prep Time: 10 minutes Cook Time: 0 minutes Servings: 2**

## Ingredients

- 1 cup of rolled oats
- 1 cup of mixed berries
- 1 banana, sliced
- 1 cup of almond milk or any milk of your choice
- 1/2 cup of Greek yogurt (plain or vanilla)
- 1 tbsp honey or maple syrup (optional)
- 1/2 tsp vanilla extract (optional)
- Ice cubes

## Instructions

1. Put oats in a blender and blend them until they become powdered.
2. In that case, we must add mixed berries, banana, almond milk, Greek yogurt, honey or maple syrup and vanilla extract to the blender with the ground oats.
3. Blend well all the smoothie's ingredients. Should your smoothie be too thick, you may put more milk into it until your preferred consistency is attained. Add ice cubes (optional) to chill your smoothie if you are using fresh berries.
4. The smoothies should be poured into glasses and served immediately.

**Nutrition (Per Serving):**

Calories: 300 kcal Protein: 12 g Carbohydrates: 45 g Fats: 5 g Fiber: 6 g

# 3. Tropical Smoothie

**Prep Time: 10 minutes Cook Time: 0 minutes Servings: 2**

## Ingredients

- 1 cup of pineapple, chopped
- 1 cup of mango, chopped
- 1 banana, sliced
- 1 cup of coconut milk or almond milk
- 1/2 cup of Greek yogurt
- Juice of 1 lime
- Optional: 1 tbsp honey or agave syrup for sweetness
- Optional: 1/4 cup of ice cubes (if using fresh fruit)

## Instructions

1. Combine mango, pineapple, and banana in a blender.
2. Put coconut milk and also Greek yogurt into it. If you're using honey or agave syrup, add it now.
3. Squeeze juice from one lime.
4. Blend ingredients till smooth. If you use fresh fruit and want a cooler smoothie, put the ice cubes in it and blend it until it's smooth.
5. Serve in glasses immediately after blending.

**Nutrition (Per Serving):**

Calories: 250 kcal Protein: 7 g Carbohydrates: 40 g Fats: 5g Fiber: 4 g

# 4. Peanut Butter & Jelly Smoothie

**Prep Time: 10 minutes Cook Time: 0 minutes Servings: 2**

## Ingredients

- 2 tbsp natural peanut butter
- 1 cup of frozen mixed berries
- 1 banana, sliced
- 1 cup of almond milk or milk of choice
- 1/2 cup of Greek yogurt
- 1 tbsp honey or maple syrup (optional)
- Optional: 1 scoop of protein powder
- Ice cubes

## Instructions

1. Put peanut butter, frozen mixed berries, a banana, almond milk, Greek yogurt, honey, or maple syrup into the blender.
2. Add protein powder.
3. Blend all on high until smooth. If you prefer a thicker and colder smoothie, add some ice cubes and then blend again.
4. If it is too thick, add more milk and blend to attain the desired consistency.
5. Serve immediately by pouring into glasses.

**Nutrition (Per Serving):**

Calories: 300 kcal Protein: 10g Carbohydrates: 35 g Fats: 12 g Fiber: 5 g

# 5. Avocado Smoothie



## Ingredients

- 1 ripe avocado, peeled and pitted
- 1 banana, sliced
- 1 cup of spinach leaves
- 1 cup of almond milk or milk of choice
- 1/2 cup of Greek yogurt
- 1 tbsp honey or maple syrup
- Ice cubes
- Optional: a few mint leaves or a squeeze of lime for added flavor

## Instructions

1. To begin, blend avocado, banana, spinach (if using), almond milk, Greek yogurt and honey or maple syrup.
2. After that, it is smooth.
3. Blend at high speed until everything becomes smooth and creamy; add some more milk until the consistency is right for you.
4. If desired, put mint leaves in or squeeze a lime and blend for a few seconds.
5. Finally, pour into serving glasses and serve right away.

**Nutrition (Per Serving)**

Calories: 300 kcal Protein: 8 g Carbohydrates: 25 g Fats: 15 g Fiber: 7 g

# 6. Green Machine Smoothie

**Prep Time: 10 minutes Cook Time: 0 minutes Servings: 2**

## Ingredients

- 2 cups of fresh spinach leaves
- 1 cup of kale leaves (stems removed)
- 1 green apple, cored and chopped
- 1 ripe banana
- 1/2 cucumber, chopped
- 1 cup of unsweetened almond milk
- Juice of 1 lemon
- 1 tbsp chia seeds (optional)
- 1 tbsp honey or agave syrup
- Ice cubes

## Instructions

1. Put spinach, kale, green apple, banana, cucumber, almond milk, lemon juice and chia seeds into a blender.
2. Blend them until all the contents are combined well, and the smoothie reaches a silky consistency. If this is too thick, add a little more almond milk.
3. Add honey or agave syrup to make it sweeter, then blend again.
4. If you need a cold smoothie, throw in some ice cubes and blend them until they are completely broken down.
5. It should be poured directly into glasses and served instantly to retain maximum freshness.

**Nutrition (Per Serving)**

Calories: 200 kcal Protein: 5 g Carbohydrates: 30 g Fats: 4 g Fiber: 4 g

# 7. Keto Smoothie

**Prep Time: 5 minutes Cook Time: 0 minutes Servings: 2**

## Ingredients

- 1 cup of unsweetened almond milk
- 1/2 cup of full-fat Greek yogurt or coconut cream
- 1/4 cup of avocado, peeled and pitted
- 2 tbsp almond butter or peanut butter
- 1 tbsp cocoa powder (unsweetened)
- 1 tbsp chia seeds
- Sweetener to taste
- Ice cubes (optional)

## Instructions

1. Take a blender and put in almond milk, Greek yogurt/coconut cream, avocado, almond butter/peanut butter, cocoa powder, chia seeds and any sweetener you like.
2. Let it blend for some time until smoothness is felt. To have a cold or thicker smoothie, put ice cubes in and blend again if desired.
3. Taste the smoothie and increase or decrease the sweetness depending on your taste buds.
4. Serve immediately by pouring the smoothies into glasses.

**Nutrition (Per Serving)**

Calories: 300 kcal Protein: 10 g Carbohydrates: 6 g Fats: 20 g Fiber: 5 g

# 8. Spinach Smoothie

**Prep Time: 5 minutes Cook Time: 0 minutes Servings: 2**

## Ingredients

- 2 cups of fresh spinach leaves
- 1 ripe banana, sliced
- 1 apple, cored and chopped
- 1/2 cup of Greek yogurt
- 1 cup of almond milk or any milk of your choice
- 1 tbsp honey or maple syrup
- Ice cubes
- Optional: 1 tbsp chia seeds or flaxseeds for extra nutrition

## Instructions

1. Put the spinach leaves and almond milk in a blender and blend them until they are completely broken.
2. Slice bananas, chop apples, and add Greek yogurt and optional honey or maple syrup to the blender. Similarly, you can include chia seeds or flaxseeds if you prefer.
3. Blend all of them properly. If the mixture is too thick for your liking, use more milk for that purpose. If you want it cooler, add ice cubes and blend again.
4. Pour the smoothie into glasses and serve it immediately.

**Nutrition (Per Serving):**

Calories: 200 kcal Protein: 6 g Carbohydrates: 30 g Fats: 2 g Fiber: 5 g

# 9. Mango Smoothie

**Prep Time: 5 minutes Cook Time: 0 minutes Servings: 2**

## Ingredients

- 2 cups of ripe mango, cubed
- 1 banana, sliced
- 1 cup of Greek yogurt
- 1 cup of orange juice or almond milk
- Optional: 1 tbsp honey or agave syrup for extra sweetness
- Ice cubes

## Instructions

1. Drop the cuboid mango in a mixer; then pour banana, Greek yogurt, orange juice, or almond milk.
2. Please do it now if you use honey or agave syrup as sweeteners.
3. Put all of them on and blend them on high until smooth. Or you can put ice cubes if you have a cold smoothie with fresh mangos.
4. If the smoothie is too thick, add small amounts of juice or milk and mix well until it is perfect for drinking.
5. Now immediately serve in glasses as a refreshment.

**Nutrition (Per Serving):**

Calories: 250 kcal Protein: 6 g Carbohydrates: 45 g Fats: 2 g Fiber: 4 g

# 10. Chocolate Peanut Butter Cup Smoothie

**Prep Time: 5 minutes Cook Time: 0 minutes Servings: 2**

## Ingredients

- 2 bananas, sliced and frozen
- 2 tbsp peanut butter
- 2 tbsp cocoa powder, unsweetened
- 1 cup of almond milk or milk of choice
- 1 scoop of chocolate protein powder
- 1 tbsp honey or maple syrup
- Ice cubes

Optional toppings: whipped cream, chocolate shavings, or a sprinkle of peanut butter powder

## Instructions

1. In a blender, take the frozen bananas, peanut butter, cocoa powder, almond milk, and chocolate protein powder (optional). Add honey or maple syrup if you want it sweeter.
2. Blend until smooth. The milk may be increased if the smoothie is too thick for you. If it's too thin, add some ice cubes and blend again.
3. Then, pour it into glasses as required. Add whipped cream or shaved chocolates on top, or sprinkle some more peanut butter in powdered form to cap this off with a bit of luxury.
4. Serve right away to get the most out of its flavor and texture.

**Nutrition (Per Serving):**

Calories: 300 kcal Protein: 10 g Carbohydrates: 35 g Fats: 12 g Fiber: 5 g

# 11. Chocolate Smoothie

**Prep Time: 5 minutes Cook Time: 0 minutes Servings: 2**

## Ingredients

- 2 bananas, sliced and frozen
- 2 tbsp cocoa powder, unsweetened
- 1 cup of almond milk or milk of choice
- 1/2 cup of Greek yogurt
- 1 tbsp honey or maple syrup
- 1 tsp vanilla extract
- Ice cubes
- Optional: 1 scoop of chocolate protein powder for added protein

## Instructions

1. Combine the frozen bananas, cocoa powder, almond milk, Greek yogurt, honey or maple syrup (if desired), vanilla extract and chocolate protein powder (if using) in a blender.
2. Blend until smooth on high. If preferred, add ice cubes for a thicker texture and blend again.
3. Sample the smoothie, then sweeten it with more honey or maple syrup as necessary.
4. Serve immediately in glasses.

**Nutrition (Per Serving):**

Calories: 250 kcal Protein: 8 g Carbohydrates: 35 g Fats: 3 g Fiber: 5 g

# 12. Green Apple Smoothie

**Prep Time: 5 minutes Cook Time: 0 minutes Servings: 2**

## Ingredients

- 2 green apples, cored and chopped
- 1 banana, sliced
- 1 cup of spinach or kale leaves
- 1/2 cup of Greek yogurt (plain or vanilla)
- 1 cup of almond milk or any milk of choice
- 1 tbsp honey or maple syrup
- Ice cubes
- Optional: 1 tbsp chia seeds or flaxseeds for added nutrients

## Instructions

1. Put the diced green apples, banana, spinach or kale, Greek yogurt, almond milk and honey or maple syrup, where applicable, in a mixer. Don't forget to include chia seeds or flaxseeds if you add them.
2. Blend at high speed until all the ingredients mix thoroughly, and the mixture becomes smooth. You may add more milk if you want your smoothie to be less viscous. If you like it thicker, blend it with several ice cubes.
3. After tasting your smoothie, you can add some honey or maple syrup to make it sweeter.
4. Pour the smoothie into glasses and serve immediately for the best taste.

**Nutrition (Per Serving)**

Calories: 200 kcal Protein: 6 g Carbohydrates: 35 g Fats: 1 g Fiber: 5 g

# 13. Chocolate Banana Smoothie

**Prep Time: 5 minutes Cook Time: 0 minutes Servings: 2**

## Ingredients

- 2 ripe bananas, sliced and frozen
- 2 tbsp cocoa powder, unsweetened
- 1 cup of almond milk or any milk of your choice
- 1/2 cup of Greek yogurt
- 1 tbsp honey or maple syrup
- Ice cubes
- Optional: 1 scoop of chocolate or vanilla protein powder for added protein

## Instructions

1. If desired, place the frozen bananas, cocoa powder, almond milk, Greek yogurt, and honey or maple syrup in a blender. If using protein powder, add it to the blender, too.
2. Blend at high speed until smooth. If it is too thick, add more milk to change its thickness. Alternatively, when you prefer a thick smoothie, add ice cubes and blend again.
3. Sip your smoothie to see if there is any need for more sweetness by pouring some more honey or maple syrup.
4. Pour into glasses and serve instantly.

**Nutrition (Per Serving):**

Calories: 250 kcal Protein: 6 g Carbohydrates: 40 g Fats: 4 g Fiber: 5 g

# 14. Berry Blast Smoothie

**Prep Time: 5 minutes Cook Time: 0 minutes Servings: 2**

## Ingredients

- 1 cup of frozen mixed berries
- 1 banana, sliced
- 1/2 cup of Greek yogurt
- 1 cup of orange juice or almond milk
- Optional: 1 tbsp honey or maple syrup for added sweetness
- Optional: 1 scoop of protein powder for added protein
- Ice cubes

## Instructions

1. Combine frozen mixed berries, banana, Greek yoghurt, orange juice or almond milk and add honey or maple syrup to taste, if desired, in a blender. Add protein powder if you want.
2. Mix all the ingredients until smooth by blending on high speed. If it is too thick, add more juice or milk. If you like it even colder, mix it with the ice cubes added.
3. Try the smoothie and adjust the sweetener based on your preference.
4. Serve immediately by pouring into glasses.

**Nutrition (Per Serving):**

Calories: 200 kcal Protein: 5 g Carbohydrates: 35 g Fats: 2 g Fiber: 4 g

# 28 DAYS MEAL PLAN

| DAY | BREAKFAST | LUNCH | DINNER |
| --- | --- | --- | --- |
| 01 | Pumpkin Pancakes | Avocado and Salmon Salad | Lentil Soup |
| 02 | Avocado Toast | Italian Pasta Salad | Beef Shish Kebabs |
| 03 | Breakfast Salad | Garlic Parmesan Fries | Farfalle with Chicken and Pesto |
| 04 | Hard-Boiled Eggs with Avocado Toast | Chicken Kabobs | Mediterranean Shrimp Penne |
| 05 | Peanut Butter and Banana Sandwich | Cream of Broccoli Soup | Parmesan-Crusted Salmon |
| 06 | Keto Waffles | Macro Roast Beef | Vegetable Pasta |
| 07 | Egg White Frittata | Bourbon Lime Salmon | Vegetable Soup |
| 08 | Maple Pecan Banana Muffins | Salmon Chickpea Salad | Cabbage Slaw |
| 09 | Cherry Protein Porridge | Roasted Butternut Squash | Spicy Turkey Stir Fry |
| 10 | Homemade Scallion Hash Brown Cakes | High-Protein Spaghetti | Sweet Potato & Green Pea Soup |
| 11 | Clean Protein Power Bars | Roasted Balsamic Chicken | Bell Pasta with Kidney Beans |
| 12 | Superfood Breakfast Bowl | Shrimp Creole | Lemon-Herb Grilled Chicken Salad |
| 13 | Cottage Cheese with Fruit and Honey | Curried Chickpea Salad | Japanese Steak Curry |
| 14 | Oatmeal with Protein Powder | Garlic Mashed Sweet Potatoes | Garlic and Herb Seared Salmon |
| 15 | Breakfast Burrito | Grilled Tuna Teriyaki | Olive Chicken |
| 16 | Breakfast Smoothie | Chicken Chili | Sea Bass with Vegetables |

| 17 | Chocolate Banana Protein Pancakes | Muscle Lentil Soup | Chicken Stir-Fry |
| 18 | Greek Egg Scramble | Traditional Shrimp Scampi | Italian Tuna Salad |
| 19 | Banana Pancakes | Pork Loin with Baked Apples | Lentil and Feta Tabbouleh |
| 20 | Breakfast Bake | Tangy Trout | Brawny Baked Haddock with Spinach |
| 21 | Asparagus and Swiss Cheese Frittata | Summer Squash Casserole | Salad with Grilled Chicken |
| 22 | Egg and Cheese Muffins | Lemon Dill Salmon | Low-Fat Chicken Bacon Ranch Sandwich |
| 23 | Apple Cinnamon Oatmeal | Grilled Chicken Breast Sandwich | Whole Wheat Pasta with Marinara Sauce |
| 24 | Scrambled Eggs with Black Beans and Salsa | Spicy Buffalo Macaroni and Cheese | Shrimp Taco Salad |
| 25 | Banana Bread Muffins | Lentil Stew | Cilantro Lime Low-Carb Rice |
| 26 | Greek Yogurt with Berries and Nuts | Classic Steak | Avocado and Tuna Salad |
| 27 | Hash Browns with Eggs | Shrimp Shiitake Pot Stickers | Citrus Spinach |
| 28 | Avocado & Egg Toast | Stuffed Mushrooms | Salmon with Quinoa and Roasted Veggies |